FULFILLING THE ESSENCE

FULFILLING THE ESSENCE

A Handbook of Traditional & Contemporary Chinese Treatments for Female Infertility

Bob Flaws

Blue Poppy Press   Boulder, CO

Published by:

BLUE POPPY PRESS
1775 LINDEN AVE.
BOULDER, CO 80304

FIRST EDITION, SEPTEMBER 1993

ISBN 0-936185-48-1
LC 93-72798

COPYRIGHT 1993 © BLUE POPPY PRESS

Printed at Westview Press, Boulder, CO on acid free, recycled paper.
Cover printed at C & M Press, Thornton, CO.

Council of Oriental Medical Publishers (COMP) Categorization: Original work and functionally translated compilation

10 9 8 7 6 5 4 3 2 1

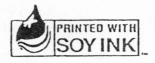

Preface

Female infertility is categorized as a *za bing* or miscellaneous disease in Chinese *fu ke* or gynecology texts. Previously I have written textbooks on the other four major clinical specialties within traditional Chinese gynecology: *My Sister the Moon* on menstrual diseases, *Fire in the Valley* on abnormal vaginal discharges and diseases of the external genitalia, and *Path of Pregnancy, Vol. I & II* on pre- and postpartum diseases. Of the other *fu ke za bing*, I have covered mastitis and uterine prolapse in Vol. II of *Path of Pregnancy*. Plum seed qi and agitated viscera are today, for political reasons, more properly discussed under *shen jing jing shen ke* or neurology/psychiatry, and abdominal masses are perhaps best left to the *zhong liu ke* or tumor specialist. Of the traditional *fu ke za bing*, infertility is the one which, over the last dozen years, I have been called upon to treat again and again. As of this writing, the treatment of female infertility comprises about 25% of my practice.

This book began, as so many of my other publications, as my own research. Treating women suffering from infertility on a regular basis, I have met with many difficult cases which have caused me to translate all the Chinese language literature available to me on this subject and pour over everything else available in English. This research has, in large part, been spurred by the paucity and incompleteness of the existing English language TCM literature on this subject. Often when treating patients, I have felt I was working with only fragments of what is necessary to do a professionally competent job. This is especially so since the treatment of infertility is emotionally unlike the treatment of any other disease.

In the treatment of infertility, there are no partial cures as is so often the case in other areas of medicine. In general clinical practice, complete and total cures of chronic diseases are the exception rather than the rule. Nonetheless, we can almost always alleviate some measure of the patient's discomfort or cure a portion of their complaints. But in infertility, the patient's goal is to get pregnant and give birth to a healthy baby. Nothing less than that is truly acceptable. And, not only is complete fulfillment of this goal the only measure of success, often treatment must span 6-15 months with a monthly report card in the form of the menses and an insistently ticking biological clock. Thus the treatment of female infertility is fraught with great emotional stress for both the patient and her TCM practitioner.

However, there are few things in clinical practice as gratifying as being responsible, at least in part, for the birth of a child. Once I visited the office of a *lao yi sheng* or old Chinese doctor in Oakland, Henry Wong. In his waiting room were scrapbooks of testimonials from satisfied and grateful patients. Most of these, it seemed, included pictures of healthy, happy children whom the loving parents credited to the skill of Dr. Wong. What a wonderful record of a physician's life work!

More women seek treatment from TCM practitioners in general than men. Surveys have shown that the age group making the most use of TCM in the United States is the baby boom generation, the oldest of whom have reached their mid-40s. Members of this generation have often postponed marriage until their 30s and begin trying to have children relatively late. In addition, this same group's diet has been mostly quite poor, our levels of work and emotional stress are generally quite high, and we have been exposed to a great deal of iatrogenesis, pollutants, and toxins. Therefore, it is no wonder that many women seeking TCM treatment in the West complain of infertility.

When TCM successfully treats female infertility, it does so comparatively inexpensively and without iatrogenesis. Since TCM is a holistic medicine, its treatments result in improving the patient's entire state of being. However, both technically and emotionally, treating infertility is no easy matter and Western TCM practitioners need all the help we can get. Because of differences in our societies, Western women seeking treatment for infertility tend to be older than Chinese women seeking treatment for the same problem. Since age is directly related to fertility in women, our patient population is more difficult to treat for that reason alone. Therefore, I have decided to share with the profession the fruits of my research in this field to date. Although I am sure there is much, much more to this subject, I hope this small addition to the English language literature helps both practitioners and patients alike achieve the miraculous goal of bringing a new life into the world.

As we all know, it takes two to tango. When a couple complains of infertility, both partners must be tested to identify where the problem lies. According to *The Merck Manual*, in 40% of couples seeking treatment for infertility, the problem lies with the man. As a specialist in TCM gynecology, my own expertise is limited to treating infertility in females and this book only deals with that half of the equation. *A Handbook of Traditional Chinese Urology & Male Sexual Dysfunction* written by Anna Lin and published by Blue Poppy Press discusses the treatment of male infertility by TCM. Those practitioners wishing to treat both male and female infertility patients should refer to that book when treating men.

Traditional Chinese Medicine in China these days is undergoing many changes due to the influence of modern Western medicine. As the reader will see, this is especially apparent in the field of infertility. This book covers both the traditional theory and treatment of infertility and also describes the most modern advances in Chinese TCM treatment utilizing Western disease categories and biological knowledge. Because of this amalgamation of traditional Chinese and modern Western knowledge, the practitioner is advised to become conversant with Western reproductive anatomy and physiology. Personally, I find this union of Eastern and Western medicine exciting, and, when approached cautiously and systematically, my experience is that it can result in hybrid vigor. In any case, there is much for contemporary practitioners to learn when they choose to treat infertility. Hopefully this book will help in that learning.

As in other recent Blue Poppy Press publications, I have tried to use Wiseman and Boss' terminology throughout. Readers unfamiliar with this terminology should see their *Glossary of Chinese Medical Terms and Acupuncture Points*. Formulas are identified by their Pinyin names. Individual medicinals are first identified in Latinate pharmacological nomenclature followed by Pinyin in parentheses. Identifications are based on Bensky and Gamble's *Chinese Herbal Medicine: Materia Medica*, Hong-yen Hsu's *Oriental Materia Medica: A Concise Guide*, Stuart and Read's *Chinese Materia Medica*, and the *Zhong Yao Da Ci Dian (An Encyclopedia of Chinese Herbs)*. In the few instances where I have not been able to make a positive identification, I have given the Pinyin followed by the Chinese characters in parentheses. Hopefully this will allow others with greater resources or knowledge to identify these ingredients.

No amounts have been specified for the ingredients of the formulas contained herein since these must be decided on an *ad hoc* basis in clinical practice. Likewise, the reader is cautioned that the formulas contained in this book are mere guides to prescribing and must be tailored to each individual patient by adding and subtracting ingredients as necessary. The reader will find the sources of the information in this book listed in the bibliography at the back. This is divided into Chinese and English language sources.

Since approximately 30 TCM journals are published every 1-2 months in the People's Republic of China and the treatment of female infertility is one of the most common topics discussed in these journals, practitioners interested in this field are strongly encouraged to begin attempting to read these journals. The movement towards the integration of TCM and modern Western medicine has only just begun, and I am sure many new protocols will be developed over the coming years which will be published in these journals. Hopefully, this book gives a good idea of the state of the art at the present time. However, if it piques the interest of other Western practitioners to find out for themselves what these 30 bimonthly journals contain and if, on that basis, they begin trying to learn to read medical Chinese, this book will have served an even greater purpose.

Bob Flaws
April, 1993

Contents

1

Modern Western Medicine & Infertility

Eighty percent of couples having regular sex without contraception will conceive within one year with another 10% conceiving after that. This suggests that around 10% of the population suffers from infertility. Of this number, 40% is due to female problems, 40% to male problems, and 10% to a combination of both acting synergistically. Peak fertility seems to occur between 21-25 years of age in both males and females after which it gradually declines. After 25 years of age, there is a 75% chance of pregnancy within 6 months. Approaching 30, this decreases to only a 47% chance. Approaching 40, this further decreases to only a 25% chance, and after 40 to a 22% chance. Another way of stating these statistics is that a woman's risk of infertility is 2 times greater in women between 35 and 44 than in women between 30 and 34. It also seems that the risk of infertility is 1½ times higher for African Americans than for whites. In China, primary infertility is defined as failure to conceive after two years of having regular sex without contraception. Secondary infertility refers to a woman who is not able to conceive for two years of unprotected sex but who previously has been pregnant at least once.

If a couple are having unprotected sex on a regular basis at the right time of the menstrual cycle and the male is not at fault, there are a number of causes for female infertility. These are summarized by the outline below, taken from *The Merck Manual*.

I. Disorders of the reproductive organs

    A. Ovaries

        1. Dysgenesis, *i.e.*, defective ovarian development in utero
        2. Infection
        3. Polycystic ovarian syndrome (Stein-Leventhal syndrome)
        4. Damage due to radiation

    B. Fallopian tubes

        1. Absence
        2. Obstruction
        3. Salpingitis, *i.e.*, inflammation of the tubes
        4. Endometriosis

    C. Cervix

        1. Displacement
        2. Cervicitis
        3. Stenosis, *i.e.*, too narrow an aperture

II. Vaginitis & sexually transmitted disease

    A. Mycoplasmosis
    B. Chlamydiasis

III. Endocrine dyscrasia, *i.e.*, hormonal imbalance

    A. Pituitary failure
    B. Thyroid disturbance
    C. Adrenal hyperplasia
    D. Luteal phase defect
    E. Cervical mucous problems due to insufficient estrogen

IV. Systemic disease (*e.g.*, diabetes mellitus)

V. Genetic disorders

   A. Chromosomal abnormalities
   B. Testicular feminization syndrome

VI. Immunologic causes (*e.g.*, antisperm antibodies)

Of these, the most commonly encountered in my experience are endocrine dysfunction resulting in either failure to ovulate or luteal phase defect, endometriosis, obstruction of the fallopian tubes, polycystic ovarian syndrome, and antisperm antibodies.

The Menstrual Cycle

For the purposes of this book and based on the Chinese infertility literature, we will divide the menstrual cycle into four phases. These we will refer to as phase I, the proliferative phase; phase II, the ovulatory phase; phase III, the postovulatory or luteal phase; and phase IV, menstruation. Modern Western reproductive endocrinology only recognizes three phases to the menstrual cycle. In this case, the preovulatory follicular phase of Western medicine includes menstruation itself and the endometrial proliferation phase.

When counting the days of the menstrual cycle, one always begins with the onset of normal bleeding. This becomes day 1 and every subsequent day until the onset of the next period is counted from there. Therefore, for the purposes of this book, phase I refers to the 6-10th days of the cycle; phase II to the 11-16th days; phase III to the 17-28th days; and phase IV to the 1-5th days.

Beginning on day 1, the first day of normal menstruation, luteinizing hormone-releasing factor (LHF) is secreted by the hypothalamus. This stimulates the anterior pituitary to secrete follicle-stimulating hormone

(FSH). This hormone then stimulates the ovaries to develop the growth of a cohort of between 3 and 30 follicles consisting of oocytes and their surrounding cells. One to two days later, the same LHF from the hypothalamus stimulates the anterior pituitary to release luteinizing hormone (LH). These two hormones, FSH and LH, stimulate the growth and development of one of the oocytes into an ovum or egg. The other oocytes degenerate and typically fail to produce a mature egg.

Around day 5 or so and corresponding to roughly the end of the period, estrogen and particularly estradiol or E_2 secreted from the ovaries begins to increase. This estradiol stimulates progressive proliferation of the endometrial lining, thus preparing the uterus for the implantation of a fertilized ovum. Because of this, the Chinese literature refers to phase I as the proliferative phase. This proliferative phase stimulated by estrogen production and release corresponds to our phase I.

In phase II or the ovulatory phase, estrogen levels continue to rise and then accelerate and peak just before there occurs a massive, preovulatory surge of LH by the pituitary gland. In turn, just before this LH surge, progesterone secreted by the ovaries also begins to increase significantly. At roughly the same time, FSH levels decrease. The LH surge usually lasts from 36-48 hours and is composed of several large bursts of LH release. This causes the mature ovum to be released by the ovary some time 16-32 hours after the onset of this surge.

In phase III, the luteal phase, the corpus luteum of the ovary formed from the site where the ovary was released itself releases progesterone. The endometrium, under the influence of this progesterone becomes increasingly vascularized. During this time, the ovum is traveling through the fallopian tubes towards the uterus. If this ovum becomes fertilized, it will attach itself to the walls of the endometrium. However, if it does not, both E_2 and progesterone decline during the later stages of phase III and the endometrium becomes increasingly edematous. Eventually the endometrial stroma become necrotic and the endometrial lining is sloughed. This is accompanied by endometrial bleeding and the period begins. Thus begins phase IV and this cycle repeats itself with a rise in LH and FSH.

Thus it can be seen from the above brief outline of female reproductive endocrinology that normal reproductive function requires a complex interplay of endocrine glands secreting hormones which then have an effect on target organs in the body. Although the pituitary gland appears to be the central command post orchestrating this complex interplay, in fact, the pituitary itself is, among other factors, affected by mental/emotional events. Cerebral cortical function can, via the hypothalamus, have an impact on pituitary function and, therefore, reproductive endocrine secretions. Likewise, diet can have a large impact on reproductive humors. Certain foods can lead to or aggravate hyperestrogenosis which can then throw the entire luteal phase of the above cycle out of kilter. And further, as we will see below, due to the interdependence of the mind, endocrine system, and immune system, dysbiosis of the large intestine can also negatively impact on endocrine function.

Modern Western Medicine's Diagnostic Evaluation of Female Infertility

If a woman goes to a Western fertility specialist complaining of infertility and her husband's sperm are not at fault, she can expect two basic investigations. The first set of tests is to establish whether or not her ovaries are functioning normally. First of all, she will probably be asked to chart her basal body temperature (BBT) for at least 3 menstrual cycles. This is accomplished by taking one's temperature first thing every morning before getting out of bed or engaging in any activity. The thermometer used must register in tenths of a degree and it should be kept in the mouth for 3-5 minutes. The resulting temperature is then plotted on a graph corresponding to the days of the woman's cycle.

If the woman is ovulating, one should expect to see a basic biphasic graph. During menstruation and the proliferative phase, the basal body temperature or BBT should be between 0.5-1.0°F lower than after ovulation. That means between 97.2-97.4°F. After ovulation, the temperature should climb to over 98.0°F. This rise may be preceded by a 0.1-0.2°F drop just prior to ovulation. In fact, the temperature begins to climb only after ovulation has taken place and does so in response to hormones secreted by the corpus luteum an inflammation at the site of egg release. Just before menstruation, the BBT drops again, signalling the immanent onset of menstruation.

If there is no rise in temperature, this suggests failure to ovulate. While if the temperature rises but then drops back down in less than 10 days or only crawls up slowly or erratically, this suggests a luteal phase defect in progesterone production. If ovulation occurs but progesterone is insufficient, even if there is fertilization, the zygote will not implant successfully. Typically with such a luteal phase defect, one experiences an early period. On the other hand, if the postovulatory temperature remains elevated for more than 18 days, this suggests the woman is pregnant.

The second test for normal ovarian function is the so-called postcoital test. Just after ovulation is supposed to have occurred, the couple are asked to have unprotected sex. The cervical mucous is then examined within 2-16 hours of intercourse. In this way, one can check for adequate numbers of viable sperm, the consistency and pH of the cervical mucous, and can determine if ovulation has indeed taken place. If the mucous is too thin and watery, this may be due to hyperestrogenosis. If a ferning pattern due to crystallization is not seen in the cervical mucous under microscopic examination, this suggests that ovulation has not taken place. A too acidic cervical mucous which can kill sperm may be due to infection. If the sperm are found to be clumped together and dead or dying, this may be due to agglutinating antibodies to the man's sperm being produced by the woman's immune system. This is basically an allergic reaction to the foreign proteins in the man's sperm.

Another method of determining if ovulation has occurred is to draw blood and measure plasma levels of progesterone. Levels 5ng/ml or above are consistent with ovulation. This method can also be used to detect or confirm a luteal phase defect with a progesterone deficiency.

Typically, all three of these methods are used together to more reliably confirm that a woman is ovulating normally. If all three of these methods are still inconclusive, serial ultrasonography of the ovarian follicles may be employed. This means tracking the developing follicle day by day with ultrasound to see whether it matures and ruptures releasing an egg.

If the above tests confirm that ovulation is taking place, that there is no luteal phase progesterone deficiency, and that the cervical mucous and the woman's immune system are not hostile to the man's sperm, the second group of tests are used to investigate functional and anatomical competence permitting union of sperm and egg. These tests include hystosalpingogram and laparoscopy.

A hystosalpingogram is the introduction of a dye carried by the medium of salt water under pressure into the woman's uterus which is then forced into the fallopian tubes. An x-ray is taken which shows the progression of this salt water through the tubes. If this gets to the ovaries, it shows that the tubes are open and unobstructed. Thus the egg should be able to unite with the sperm and travel down to the uterus to implant.

Laparoscopy consists of making a surgical incision in the abdomen and introducing a fiber optic viewer into the abdomen. In this way, the physician can see the abdominal contents, including the ovaries, uterus, and tubes. This technique can identify obstructions to the tubes, such as adhesions or endometriosis. Often this procedure is accompanied by biopsy and laser surgery. Thus endometrial tissue can be identified and even vaporized without leaving behind further obstructive scar tissue.

7

Modern Western Medicine's Treatment of Female Infertility

Modern Western medicine typically treats mechanical obstructions to fertilization and implantation, such as endometriosis, adhesions, myomas, and fibromas, surgically. Although surgery is not bad *per se*, it is invasive, painful, requires a recuperation period, and is fraught with a certain amount of risk.

Ovulatory dysfunction due to endocrine dyscrasia is treated with hormone therapy using synthetic hormones to supply whatever is deficient or missing. This therapy is also not bad *per se* but can result in unwanted multiple pregnancies, is not always effective, and can wind up imbalancing a woman's endocrine balance even worse than before she started. Such further iatrogenic dyscrasia is because modern Western medicine has nothing comparable to *bian zheng lun zhi* or treatment based on a patient's individualized pattern. Thus the theoretically right medicine may be given to the practically-speaking wrong woman.

If infertility is due to infections of the reproductive tract causing, for instance, hostile mucous, these are treated with antibiotics. However, because beneficial commensal bacteria, yeast and fungi, and protozoa all maintain a synergistic symbiotic relationship both between themselves and their host, indiscriminately killing bacteria may have a long-term ill-effect on the patient's immune and, therefore, endocrine function.

If surgery, hormone therapy, and antibiotics fail to remedy the woman's infertility, even more sophisticated technological interventions are used. These are invasive, expensive, and frequently less than emotionally satisfactory. They include artificial insemination, *in vitro* fertilization, gamete intrafallopian transfer, frozen embryo intrafallopian transfer, and surrogate motherhood. Artificial insemination means taking the father-to-be's live, fresh sperm and mechanically introducing it into the uterus past the cervix. *In vitro* fertilization is used with women whose tubes do not permit normal passage of the fertilized zygote. An egg is surgically extracted from the ovary. It is fertilized outside the body by the father-to-be's sperm and then reintroduced into the uterus. Gamete intrafallopian transfer (GIFT) consists of extracting oocytes, fertilizing them outside the woman's body and reintroducing them into the fallopian tubes. ZIFT, zygote intrafallopian transfer, means doing the same thing with frozen embryos which are stored for use until necessary. And surrogate motherhood consists of artificially inseminating, with the father-to-be's sperm, another woman who agrees to carry the resulting fetus to term and surrender it to the infertile couple upon birth.

Ethical and legal problems abound with all these procedures. They are extremely expensive and even though they are high tech, state-of-the-art, they do not always work. In addition, these procedures have a strong psychological impact on most couples undergoing them. As the authors of *The Merck Manual* state,

> Since conception is so complex, for those couples attempting to correct their infertility, the remedial process can stretch over years and be not only an extreme financial burden, but a cause of great emotional stress... Many couples find the testing process intrusive and degrading, feeling exposed during this most intimate aspect of their lives.[1]

As mentioned above, because there is such a strong connection between the central nervous system, the hypothalamus, pituitary, and ovarian function, stress itself can mitigate against fertility. Therefore, the more stressful a remedial procedure or methodology is, the more it is working against itself.

---

[1] *The Merck Manual*, Robert Bukow, ed., Merck Sharp and Dohme Research Laboratories, Rahway, NJ, 1987, p. 1666-1667

Age and Infertility

According to the American Department of Health and Human Services, the number of women in the United States who had their first baby between the ages of 30-39 doubled in the period from 1970-1986. In the Netherlands, the average age of primiparas is 27.6 years and in Belgium it is 26.2 years. Professor te Velde of the University of Utrecht states that:

> The postponement of the first pregnancy is clearly linked to the progress of women's emancipation. The emancipation process was boosted when reliable contraception, such as the Pill, became available on a large scale. The considerable improvement in contraceptive methods has also enabled more and more women to enter the workforce.[2]

Professor Devroey of the Center for Reproductive Medicine at the Free University in Brussels further explains:

> In contemporary women, the wish to become a mother manifests itself at a later phase in life. In some cases, this desire expresses a fear of lacking something very essential in life. The increase in the number of older women desiring a child may also be related to the increased divorce rate. A new couple often considers a child as the fulfillment of their relationship.[3]

Certainly it is my experience as a clinician working in the United States that most of my infertility patients are between the ages of 35-42. However, the postponement of child-bearing in industrialized countries has its down side and inevitable consequences. One study suggests that the critical age at which fertility diminishes is 31 years

---

[2] *Orgyn*, te Velde, E. R., quoted by Henk Hellema, "To Conceive or Not to Conceive," The Netherlands, Vol. IV, No. 1, 1993, p. 4

[3] Devroey, P., quoted by Henk Hellema, *op. cit.*, p. 4

old. According to this study, fertility diminishes gradually, but at 35, the monthly chance of pregnancy is only half that of what it was at 30. And at 38, it is only half of what it was at 35. Western researchers think that the most important factor of diminished fertility in women over 30 is the aging of their ovae.

It is ironic that at the time when women are becoming most impatient to conceive, conception typically takes so much longer. Devroey and te Velde believe that women should be made more aware that pregnancy is increasingly difficult to achieve once a woman has passed 30 years of age. I agree that Western women need to be educated to the fact that delaying child-bearing past the early 30s at the most may result in never having a biological child at all. In my experience, too many Western women believe that having a baby in their mid to late 30s or even into their 40s is easily possible. In fact, women who think this way run the very real risk of not being able to get and stay pregnant when they finally decide the time is right. I agree with te Velde when he says:

> We shall have to accept the fact that it is not possible for women to achieve their career goals in the same way men do. This means that fitting regulations should be set up for matters such as parental leave and child care.[4]

Many women's assumptions about child-bearing in their 30s and 40s are based on ignorance of the true facts about female fertility and age. On the one hand, in order to stem the rising tide of frustrated couples with fertility problems, researchers and clinicians need to get this information out to the public. On the other, we as societies in the industrialized West need to enact social programs so women can have a career and have children *at the same time.*

---

[4] te Velde, *Ibid.*, p. 5

2

Traditional Chinese Medicine & Infertility

Traditional Chinese Medicine (TCM) provides a low cost, noninvasive, and noniatrogenic alternative and complement to modern Western medicine in the treatment of female infertility. Because TCM focuses on rebalancing individuals and not just treating diseases, its treatments are tailor-made and have low potential for iatrogenesis or side effects. In addition, they tend to promote the systemic health and well being of the entire person. This being the case, it makes sense to first attempt to correct female infertility through TCM and then, if that fails, to subsequently employ the more forceful but also more risky treatments of modern Western medicine. It is also possible to use the high tech diagnostic tests of modern Western medicine and its pathophysiological specificity in tandem with the holistic, benign, but nonetheless effective therapies of TCM.

The TCM Theory of Fertility & Conception

The foundations of Chinese medicine were developed more than 2,000 years ago, well before the invention of the microscope. Therefore, there are many biological facts which were unknown to those doctors who laid the theoretical basis of TCM. Chinese doctors knew that women only conceive after menarche and before menopause. They knew that the male had to ejaculate within the vagina of the female and they could see the ejaculate with their naked eyes. However, the only things they saw coming out of the healthy female vagina were the menses and babies. They also knew that when a woman becomes pregnant her menses typically ceases. Therefore, they were able to make a connection between fertility and the period.

In fact, although TCM theory says that the reproductive essence of both male and female, the *sheng zhi zhi jing*, must unite in the womb for fertilization to take place, Chinese doctors, not being able to see the egg, have traditionally identified this female reproductive essence with the woman's menstrual blood. Fu Qing-zhu, the single most famous Chinese gynecologist in history, said:

> ...the menstruation is not blood but heavenly water or the *tian gui*. Originating in the kidneys, it is the essence of consummate yin (the kidneys), but possessed of the qi of consummate yang (the heart). Therefore, it is red like blood but it is, in fact, not blood. This accounts for its name, the *tian gui* or heavenly water.

Therefore, in TCM it is the union of the red essence of the woman with the white essence of the man which forms the zygote. If the white essence of the man is ejaculated into the womb of a post-menarche woman, there can be two basic reasons why conception does not take place. Either this red essence is insufficient in supply or something is blocking it from uniting with the man's *sheng zhi zhi jing*.

Bing Li
Pathophysiology

Historically, Chao Yuan-fang of the Sui Dynasty (589-618 CE), in his book, *Zhu Bing Yuan Hou Lun (Treatise on Various Diseases and the Source of their Symptoms)*, said that female infertility is due to cold evil qi settling in the *jing* (channels/menses) and blood. In the Song Dynasty (960-1280 CE), in the *Sheng Ji Zong Lu (The Imperial Collection & Record of Aid)*, it says that if there is kidney qi vacuity cold, the uterus will not be able to be tied up. Zhu Dan-xi of the Jin-Yuan (1280-1368 CE), in his book, *Dan Xi Xin Fa (Dan-xi's Heart Methods)*, said, "(If) a person's body is packed and overflowing with fat or grease, this may block and obstruct the uterus." In other words, over the centuries, different Chinese doctors have advanced a number of reasons why women may be infertile. In modern TCM, all these causes are considered and taken into account. However, in order to understand these historical and somewhat cryptic accounts of female infertility, a fuller discussion of female reproduction and the disease causes and mechanisms associated with problems in reproduction is necessary.

TCM posits the existence of two types of essence or *jing*. The first is called the *xian tian zhi jing*. This is normally translated as the prenatal essence but more literally means the before heaven essence. Before heaven here refers to a metaphysical/cosmological concept in Chinese philosophy. This *xian tian zhi jing* is associated with and stored in the kidneys. It is in charge of the person's constitution, maturation and decline, and reproduction. In terms of the blood or female essence, we can say that this kidney *jing* provides the substrate or foundation of the woman's blood essence. The second type of essence is called the *hou tian zhi jing*. Commonly translated as postnatal essence but more properly referred to as the after heaven essence, this is also called the acquired essence. It is manufactured from the surplus qi and blood left after a day's activities. This qi and blood are in turn derived from the finest essence of food and liquids consumed by the stomach and transformed by the spleen. Therefore, the spleen and stomach are often referred to as the *hou tian zhi ben* or postnatal root. It is this acquired essence and especially the blood generated and transformed by the spleen which amplifies and makes robust the female reproductive essence.

According to the *Su Wen*, at 2 times 7, or 14 years of age, the kidneys are flourishing, the *chong mai* is full of blood, the *ren mai* is open and patent, and the female is able to conceive. This flourishing of the kidneys is due, in large part, to the maturation of the spleen/stomach or digestion and the robust creation postnatally of blood and acquired essence. Therefore, in terms of blood production, although it is said that the heart turns the blood red, *i.e.*, participates in the final transformation and generation of blood, the two main organs discussed in modern TCM texts *vis à vis* female fertility are the kidneys and spleen.

Although kidney *jing* is comparatively yin to qi's being yang, essence itself holds within it the seeds of both yin and yang. This means that it can be transformed into yin substance or yang qi as necessary. Therefore, either kidney yin vacuity or kidney yang vacuity may be associated with insufficient *jing* and blood. Kidney yin vacuity may be due to constitutional insufficiency, chronic disease, overtaxation, excessive sex, drug abuse, aging, or chronic malnutrition. If there is insufficient kidney yin, yang typically comes out of balance and control. If yang becomes pathologically effulgent, vacuity heat results. This scorches and evaporates blood and yin fluids and can result in further insufficiency of blood and yin.

On the other hand, because of constitutional weakness and debility, chronic disease, malnutrition, excessive sex, drug abuse, aging, and overtaxation, a person may also suffer from kidney yang vacuity. Since kidney yang or *yuan* source qi is the motivating force for all transformations in the body, blood may not be produced abundantly. Further, because kidney yang is the source of warmth in the lower burner and life and growth are warm, there may be insufficient warmth to maintain and foster an embryo. And, since kidney yang also keeps blood and body fluids flowing freely in the pelvis, kidney yang vacuity may result in impeded or retarded blood flow in the uterus as well.

Han Bai-ling says that abortions and habitual miscarriage harm the kidneys, although he does not say exactly how or whether yin or yang: "If (the patient) has had any abortions or has suffered from habitual miscarriage followed by infertility, these punish the kidneys and treatment cannot be mistaken."

In terms of viscera and bowels, it is the liver which treasures or stores the blood. The liver is the child of the kidneys according to five phase theory. Since blood and essence are so closely identified in women, it is sometimes said that the liver is the before heaven viscera in a woman. It is also said that the liver and kidneys share a common source, this source being the *jing* essence. Therefore, if either kidney yin or yang vacuity results in insufficient essence, it often results in liver blood vacuity as well. Since blood is the mother of qi, if liver blood becomes scant, liver qi can become congested. Since it is qi which moves the blood, over time blood stasis may further complicate this scenario.

As we have seen above, the spleen plays a major role in the generation and transformation of blood from the finest essence of food and liquids. If the spleen becomes weak through overtaxation, worry, or faulty diet, such as overeating too sweet food or overeating cold, raw foods, the spleen may lose its ability to generate and transform the blood. Since the spleen is also the postnatal root of qi production and qi is the commander of the blood, qi vacuity may result in an inability to hold the blood within the *jing* channels. Pathologic bleeding, such as early or excessive periods, thus results in a further reduction in blood and body fluids.

Further, the spleen is responsible for transporting and transforming water in the body. If the spleen becomes deficient and damaged, it may lose control over this transportation and transformation. Dampness may accumulate and, since dampness is heavy, it tends to percolate down into the lower burner, there obstructing the flow of qi and blood and hindering true yang. If dampness congeals, it may turn into phlegm and this phlegm may obstruct the channels and connecting vessels, thus hindering and blocking the flow of blood to and through the uterus.

Emotional frustration and stress may also cause liver qi. As mentioned above, the qi commands the blood. In part this means the qi is responsible for moving the blood. It is the liver which as a viscera is responsible for ensuring coursing and discharge, including the patency of qi. If, due to emotional stress, liver depression gives rise to qi stagnation, this may block the free flow of blood to the uterus. If this qi stagnation is severe or continues long enough, it will eventually result in blood stasis causing even more serious blockage and obstruction.

Blood stasis may also be due to physical trauma to the pelvis, including surgery and artificial abortion. It may be due to invasion by evil cold from the outside, in which case evil cold constricts and congeals the blood in the pelvis. It may be due to iatrogenesis from IUDs and oral contraceptives, and may evolve from chronic inflammation. As we have seen above, phlegm dampness may be generated due to faulty spleen function and this may obstruct the free flow of qi and blood in the pelvis. If serious enough, it can give rise to blood stasis. Conversely, long term blood stasis is usually complicated by phlegm stasis since the blood, body fluids, and qi are all interdependent and flow together.

Liver depression and qi stagnation may evolve into transformative or depressive heat. This heat may stew the juices giving rise to damp heat. Dampness from faulty spleen function and improper diet may impede the free flow of the liver channel in the lower burner. The qi may become hindered and accumulate behind and within this dampness. This may likewise result in damp heat. Certain foods can also cause damp heat on their own, such as fatty greasy foods, spicy foods, alcohol, and milk products. And finally, damp heat may invade from the outside. Most sexually transmitted diseases are categorized as externally invading damp heat evils. If such externally invading damp heat evils enter the blood *fen,* their heat may waste yin and blood over time. Since heat travels upwards in the body, the heat associated with damp heat tends to also collect in the lungs and heart. In the heart, it disturbs the spirit, disrupts the heart's participation in the creation of the blood, and can disrupt the heart's sending of the blood downward to the uterus.

Whether heat precedes dampness, dampness precedes heat, or both arise in conjunction, damp heat in the lower burner may mutually wrestle and bind or knot with qi stagnation and blood stasis. Since damp heat in the large intestine can impede the source of transformation of the kidneys, damp heat in the lower burner can paradoxically also result in kidney yang vacuity and all its attendant ills.

Li Dong-yuan, in his monumental *Pi Wei Lun (Treatise on the Spleen & Stomach)*, refers to damp heat as yin fire. The heat from this yin fire easily enters the *chong mai* and the *xue fen* or blood level. Because the *chong mai* connects with the heart and also because the heart rules the blood, heat entering the *chong mai/xue fen* typically disturbs the *shen* spirit and, in women, causes various menstrual irregularities. The four most important vessels associated with menstruation are the *chong* and *ren*, *du* and *dai*. The *chong* and *ren* govern menstruation and conception, while the *du* and *ren* govern the periodicity of the cycle. According to Li, the heat associated with yin fire or damp heat may pass from the *chong* into the *du mai* and counterflow upward. As it does so, it typically also passes over into the foot *tai yang*. From there, it may fail to descend down the *ren* and congest and cause chaos in either the neck and shoulders, head and face, throat, chest, or abdomen.

The well-known *lao yi sheng*, Huang Shou-ren, in *Huang Shou Ren Yi Jing (Huang Shou-ren's Looking Glass of Medicine)*, says that the *bao gong* or uterus is governed by the two vessels of the *chong* and *ren* and that these are divided and pertain to the liver and kidneys respectively. This underscores that the liver and kidneys are intimately involved in this yin fire scenario described by Li Dong-yuan. In addition, Li sees the spleen and stomach as the pivotal organs involved in the creation of this yin fire scenario. Thus, this scenario takes into account all of the disease mechanisms described separately above, and, in my clinical experience, many Western women suffering from infertility are best described and treated keeping Li's yin fire in mind. Li's theories on the ramifications of yin fire are the best explanation I have found of the complicated mechanisms associated with many Western women's infertility.

This covers the main TCM disease causes and disease mechanisms resulting in either insufficient blood and essence or blocked blood and essence causing female infertility. These causes and mechanisms account for the eight basic patterns associated with female infertility:

kidney yang vacuity   blood stasis
kidney yin vacuity   cold uterus
blood vacuity   phlegm dampness
liver depression   damp heat

However, as we will discuss below under a separate chapter, *chong* or parasites in the form of candidiasis (*zhen jun*) may complicate a number of the above scenarios and contribute to female infertility. Further, Li Dong-yuan's theories on yin fire can provide a theoretically astute and clinically useful model of how all these disease mechanisms and their associated patterns can interact and present together.

Zhi Yuan Zhi Fa
Treatment Principles, Treatment Methods

Since the female reproductive essence is associated with the blood and the evidence of the sufficiency and patency of the female's blood essence is her monthly menstruation, it is little wonder that Zhu Dan-xi in the Jin/Yuan Dynasties said, "In order to cure infertility, the first important thing is to regulate the menstruation." This point was reemphasized by Chen Xiu-yuan in the Qing Dynasty in his *Nu Ke Yao Zhi (The Essence of Gynecology)*. Chen said, "Failure to conceive in women is always due to lack of regulation in the menstrual flow." Bick Jane Tang states this in a modern way as follows:

Female infertility frequently results from hormonal imbalance, which is expressed as problems of ovulation and anovulation. In traditional Chinese medicine, the first step in treating female infertility is regulation of the menstrual cycle which effectively regulates hormonal imbalance and induces ovulation.[1]

In Chinese medicine, *yue jing bu tiao* or lack of regulation or balance in the menstrual flow covers a number of parameters and not just periodicity. In terms of periodicity, it covers early periods, late periods, and periods which come either early or late and at no fixed intervals. However, *yue jing bu tiao* also covers irregularities in the amount, color, and consistency of the menstrual flow and any abnormal symptoms or sensations occurring in concert with menstruation, such as dysmenorrhea and premenstrual complaints. This means that *yue jing bu tiao* covers most of the disease categories covered by the *yue jing bing* or menopathy section of TCM gynecology.

The basic prescriptive methodology of modern TCM is *bian zheng lun zhi*. This means giving treatment on the basis of pattern discrimination. This is in contradistinction to basing treatment primarily on disease discrimination. When Zhang Xiao-chun says, "There are no fixed treatment measures to be followed (in the treatment of female infertility), rather one is completely reliant upon a discrimination of patterns," he means that there is no single treatment for infertility but that treatment from patient to patient must vary based on their individual patterns of disharmony. Nonetheless, based on the disease mechanisms discussed above, only certain patterns are routinely associated with infertility. Thus Han Bai-ling, one of my favorite contemporary Chinese gynecological authorities, says:

> In the Chinese medical treatment of infertility patterns, the regulation of the menstruation is of focal importance, specifically via measures for rectifying the liver, supplementing the kidneys, transforming phlegm, and, according to Wang Qing-ren, expelling

---

[1]   Tang, Bick Jane, "Traditional Chinese Herbal and Acupuncture Treatment of Female Infertility," *International Journal of Oriental Medicine*, Vol. 16, No. 2, June, 1991, p. 91

stasis. Liver depression and kidney vacuity are the most commonly observed clinical patterns.

It is assumed that if essence blood is made replete and all obstructions and hindrances to its free flow to and through the womb are cleared away, conception should take place. It is also assumed that one can know if these treatment aims have been accomplished in large part by observing the menstruation, its cyclicity, amount, color, consistency, and any accompanying signs and symptoms.

The following chapter contains a discussion of the differential diagnosis and treatment of the various patterns associated in TCM with female infertility. This discussion, although including more comprehensive treatment options than any other current TCM book on this topic, follows the pattern of most TCM *fu ke* textbooks. First there are the signs and symptoms differentiating and defining the pattern. Then there are the therapeutic principles which guide the treatment and rebalancing of the pattern. And then there are representative formulas designed to achieve those therapeutic goals.

However, in the contemporary Chinese literature, an interesting dichotomy is apparent. Most *fu ke* textbooks, even the most recent ones, all discuss the treatment of infertility according to the *bian zheng lun zhi* methodology described above. But in the Chinese TCM journals published from the mid-1980s on and in modern Chinese anthologies of case histories and compendia of effective formulas, a different approach is evident. Based on such journal articles, it is evident that there is a movement afoot in China in the treatment of infertility which is made up of three components.

First, there is an emphasis on kidney supplementation. This is based on the dictum that, "The kidneys rule reproduction (*shen zhu sheng zhi*)." No matter what other treatment principles are used, these treatments also routinely add kidney-supplementing medicinals such as Herba Epimedii (*Xian Ling Pi*), Semen Cuscutae (*Tu Si Zi*), and Radix Dipsaci (*Xu Duan*). Bick Jane Tang states:

22

Clinically, hormonal imbalance in the female is related to three internal organs: liver, spleen, and kidneys. Traditional Chinese medicine places infertility as closely related to kidney function, since the kidneys control the reproductive system.[2]

Secondly, there is an emphasis on treating named Western pathologies accounting for infertility. That means treatments are addressed to polycystic ovarian syndrome, endometriosis, blocked fallopian tubes, anovulation, and luteal phase defect rather than to infertility accompanied by early menstruation or menstrual pain. These disease-oriented approaches typically make use of the dual diagnosis favored by proponents of what is called in Chinese *zhong xi yi jie he*, combined or integrated Chinese-Western medicine. Treatment is still predicated largely on pattern discrimination but is combined with disease specific information borrowed from Western biology and Western medical diagnostic procedures.

Third, treatment is usually given along with and adjusted based on the phases of the menstrual cycle. This means that, based on certain biological facts and theoretical assumptions, different medicinals, formulas, and therapeutic principles are used during different phases of the menstrual cycle. Thus, in these modern Chinese TCM articles, differential diagnosis and treatment discriminates between disease, pattern, and menstrual cycle phase.

Personally, I have found these integrated Chinese-Western approaches to be very effective in a number of cases where a Western diagnosis has been or can be established. Chapters 4-9 below, therefore, include sample protocols from the recent Chinese journal literature. Western TCM practitioners attempting to treat infertility without access to these modern approaches which have yet to appear in standard TCM gynecology texts are severely limited in their information. It is my experience that these new protocols can spell the difference between success and failure.

---

[2]   *Ibid.*, p. 2

3

Bian Zheng Lun Zhi
Treatment According to Pattern Discrimination

The main patterns discussed in the Chinese TCM literature related to female infertility are kidney yang vacuity, kidney yin vacuity, blood vacuity, liver depression, blood stasis, cold uterus, phlegm damp accumulation and obstruction, and damp heat mutually struggling and binding with qi stagnation and blood stasis. Many TCM *fu ke* texts implicitly cover blood vacuity under liver/kidney dual vacuity. Most commonly, this refers to kidney yin and liver blood vacuity, although at least one Chinese text of which I am aware speaks of liver/kidney vacuity as meaning liver blood and kidney yang vacuity. Another Chinese TCM *fu ke* text lists qi and blood vacuity weakness as a pattern of female infertility. However, as the reader will see when studying the formulas under blood vacuity below, this nomenclature merely clarifies the relationship between the qi and blood. Some TCM gynecology books call kidney yang vacuity spleen/kidney yang vacuity. In addition, a number of Chinese texts consider cold uterus merely a subcategory of blood stasis. I have separated these out in order for practitioners to have as many different patterns as possible. Hopefully, this will enable them to categorize their patient's as precisely as possible.

I recommend that practitioners not only use the following compendium of formulas for the treatment of infertility as a source for their prescriptions but to also spend time contemplating the variations on a theme each formula under each category represents. One should strive to be able to look at any formula and, by analyzing its ingredients, immediately understand the pattern, signs, and symptoms for which the formula is most appropriate as well as the rationale for the composition of the formula. I personally feel that I have gained considerable insight into the writing of prescriptions for women suffering from infertility by collecting and studying these formulas, and I highly recommend this process to my peers.

Shen Yang Xu
Kidney Yang Vacuity

Pathognomonic manifestations: Long term infertility or infertility in an older woman, possibly a history of late menarche, delayed periods, amount scant, color pale and dull, or amenorrhea, facial color dark and dusky, low back and knee soreness and weakness, possible dizziness and/or tinnitus, poor memory, lack of warmth in the four limbs, clear, long urination, defecation not full but possibly loose, diminished sexual desire, a pale, moist tongue with thin or slimy, white coating, and a deep, thready, forceless or deep, slow pulse

Therapeutic principles: Supplement the kidneys and warm the essence, warm the yang and nourish the *bao gong*

Rx: *Yu Lin Zhu*

Radix Panacis Ginseng (*Ren Shen*)
Rhizoma Atractylodis Macrocephalae (*Bai Zhu*)
Sclerotium Poriae Cocoris (*Fu Ling*)
wine-fried Radix Albus Paeoniae Lactiflorae (*Shao Yao*)
mix-fried Radix Glycyrrhizae (*Zhi Gan Cao*)
Radix Angelicae Sinensis (*Dang Gui*)
prepared Radix Rehmanniae (*Shu Di*)
Semen Cuscutae (*Tu Si Zi*)
wine-fried Cortex Eucommiae Ulmoidis (*Du Zhong*)
Cornu Degelatinum Cervi (*Lu Jiao Shuang*)

Rhizoma Ligustici Wallichii (*Chuan Xiong*)

This formula is composed of *Si Jun Zi Tang*, *Si Wu Tang*, and ingredients to supplement the liver and kidneys, fill the essence, and supplement the eight extraordinary vessels. Shi Cheng-han, author of *Zhong Yi Fu Ke (TCM Gynecology)*, calls this pattern liver/kidney insufficiency (*gan shen bu zu*). This underscores the fact that blood vacuity typically plays a part in this pattern. Sun Jiu-ling, author of *Fu Ke Zheng Zhi (Proven Treatments in Gynecology)*, calls this pattern kidney qi deficiency detriment (*shen qi kui sun*). This emphasizes the role of qi vacuity in this condition.

Yu Lin Zhu Jia Zi He Che Dan Shen Xiang Fu

Radix Panacis Ginseng (*Ren Shen*)
Rhizoma Atractylodis Macrocephalae (*Bai Zhu*)
Sclerotium Poriae Cocoris (*Fu Ling*)
Radix Albus Paeoniae Lactiflorae (*Bai Shao*)
Rhizoma Ligustici Wallichii (*Chuan Xiong*)
mix-fried Radix Glycyrrhizae (*Zhi Gan Cao*)
Radix Angelicae Sinensis (*Dang Gui*)
prepared Radix Rehmanniae (*Shu Di*)
Semen Cuscutae (*Tu Si Zi*)
Cortex Eucommiae Ulmoidis (*Du Zhong*)
Cornu Degelatinum Cervi (*Lu Jiao Shuang*)
Fructus Zanthoxyli Bungeani (*Chuan Jiao*)
Placenta Hominis (*Zi He Che*)
Radix Salviae Miltiorrhizae (*Dan Shen*)
Rhizoma Cyperi Rotundi (*Xiang Fu*)

In this formula, Placenta Hominis is added to more forcefully supplement kidney yang and essence. Radix Salviae Miltiorrhizae is added to quicken the blood and transform stasis. And Rhizoma Cyperi Rotundi is added to rectify and move the qi.

Yu Lin Zhu Jia Jian

Radix Codonopsis Pilosulae (*Dang Shen*)
Rhizoma Atractylodis Macrocephalae (*Bai Zhu*)
Sclerotium Poriae Cocoris (*Fu Ling*)
mix-fried Radix Glycyrrhizae (*Zhi Gan Cao*)
Radix Angelicae Sinensis (*Dang Gui*)
Rhizoma Ligustici Wallichii (*Chuan Xiong*)
prepared Radix Rehmanniae (*Shu Di*)
stir-fried Radix Albus Paeoniae Lactiflorae (*Bai Shao*)
Herba Epimedii (*Xian Ling Pi*)
Semen Cuscutae (*Tu Si Zi*)
Fluoritum (*Zi Shi Ying*)
Fructus Zanthoxyli Bungeani (*Chuan Jiao*)

Shen Chong-li, author of *Zhong Yi Fu Ke Lin Chuan Shou Ce (A Handbook of Clinical TCM Gynecology)*, says to use this formula after menstruation and to use *Wen Shen Fang* during midcycle.

Wen Shen Fang

Fluoritum (*Zi Shi Ying*)
Fructus Corni Officinalis (*Shan Zhu Yu*)
Semen Cuscutae (*Tu Si Zi*)
prepared Radix Rehmanniae (*Shu Di*)
Radix Dioscoreae Oppositae (*Shan Yao*)
Sclerotium Poriae Cocoris (*Fu Ling*)
Radix Angelicae Sinensis (*Dang Gui*)
Radix Morindae Officinalis (*Ba Ji Tian*)
prepared Radix Aconiti Carmichaeli (*Shu Fu Pian*)
Rhizoma Acori Graminei (*Chang Pu*)
Cornu Cervi (*Lu Jiao Pian*)

You Gui Wan

prepared Radix Rehmanniae (*Shu Di*)
Radix Praeparatus Aconiti Carmichaeli (*Fu Zi*)
Cortex Cinnamomi (*Rou Gui*)
Fructus Corni Officinalis (*Shan Zhu Yu*)
Fructus Lycii Chinensis (*Gou Qi Zi*)
Radix Dioscoreae Oppositae (*Shan Yao*)
Cortex Eucommiae Ulmoidis (*Du Zhong*)
Radix Angelicae Sinensis (*Dang Gui*)
Semen Cuscutae (*Tu Si Zi*)
Gelatinum Cornu Cervi (*Lu Jiao Jiao*)

Jia Jian Zuo Gui Wan

prepared Radix Rehmanniae (*Shu Di*)
Radix Dioscoreae Oppositae (*Shan Yao*)
Radix Achyranthis Bidentatae (*Niu Xi*)
Fructus Corni Officinalis (*Shan Zhu Yu*)
Semen Cuscutae (*Tu Si Zi*)
Placenta Hominis (*Zi He Che*)
Fructus Lycii Chinensis (*Gou Qi*)
Gelatinum Cornu Cervi (*Lu Jiao Jiao*)
Folium Artemesiae Argyi (*Ai Ye*)
Herba Epimedii (*Yin Yang Huo*)

Wu Zi Yan Zong Wan a.k.a. Wu Zi Wan, Wu Zi Bu Shen Wan

Semen Cuscutae (*Tu Si Zi*)
Fructus Schizandrae Chinensis (*Wu Wei Zi*)
Fructus Lycii Chinensis (*Gou Qi Zi*)
Fructus Rubi (*Fu Pen Zi*)
Semen Plantaginis (*Che Qian Zi*)

This formula is given by a number of authors, including Yeung Him-che, for the treatment of kidney yang vacuity infertility. However, Du Jie-hui, author of *Nan Nu Bing Mi Yan Liang Fang (Secret, Proven, Fine Formulas for Men's & Women's Disease)*, lists it with the yin vacuity formulas or at least as a transitional formula between yin and yang vacuities. This is because several of its ingredients supplement the liver and both kidney yin and yang.

Er Si Wu He Ji

Rhizoma Curculiginis Orchoidis (*Xian Mao*)
Herba Epimedii (*Xian Ling Pi*)
Radix Angelicae Sinensis (*Dang Gui*)
Radix Albus Paeoniae Lactiflorae (*Bai Shao*)
Rhizoma Ligustici Wallichii (*Chuan Xiong*)
prepared Radix Rehmanniae (*Shu Di*)
Fructus Schizandrae Chinensis (*Wu Wei Zi*)
Semen Cuscutae (*Tu Si Zi*)
Fructus Rubi (*Fu Pen Zi*)
Fructus Lycii Chinensis (*Gou Qi Zi*)
Semen Plantaginis (*Che Qian Zi*)

This formula is a combination of the two main ingredients of *Er Xian Tang*, *Si Wu Tang*, and *Wu Zi Wan* or *Wu Zi Yan Zong Wan*.

Yi Shen Nuan Gong Tang

stir-fried Radix Codonopsis Pilosulae (*Dang Shen*)
stir-fried Rhizoma Atractylodis Macrocephalae (*Bai Zhu*)
mix-fried Radix Glycyrrhizae (*Zhi Gan Cao*)
Sclerotium Poriae Cocoris (*Fu Ling*)
Semen Cuscutae (*Tu Si Zi*)
Fructus Zanthoxyli Bungeani (*Chuan Jiao*)
Fluoritum (*Zi Shi Ying*)
Radix Angelicae Sinensis (*Quan Dang Gui*)

Fructus Rubi (*Fu Pen Zi*)
Radix Albus Paeoniae Lactiflorae (*Bai Shao*)
stir-fried Rhizoma Ligustici Wallichii (*Chuan Xiong*)
prepared Radix Rehmanniae (*Da Shu Di*)
Cornu Cervi (*Lu Jiao Pian*)
Semen Leonuri Heterophylli (*Chong Wei Zi*)

The core of this prescription is likewise made up of *Si Jun Zi Tang* and *Si Wu Tang* with ingredients to supplement the liver and kidneys, warm the uterus, and transform stasis. Shi Cheng-han says to use this formula for 7-10 days before menstruation and then to use the patent pill forms of *Ba Zhen Wan* and *Wu Zi Yan Zong Wan* after the period.

Yi Shen Yang Xue Tiao Chong Fang

Herba Epimedii (*Xian Ling Pi*)
Fluoritum (*Zi Shi Ying*)
Radix Morindae Officinalis (*Ba Ji Tian*)
Radix Dipsaci (*Xu Duan*)
Cornu Degelatinum Cervi (*Lu Jiao Shuang*)
Fructus Zanthoxyli Bungeani (*Chuan Jiao*)
Fructus Lycii Chinensis (*Gou Qi Zi*)
Radix Angelicae Sinensis (*Dang Gui*)
Rhizoma Ligustici Wallichii (*Chuan Xiong*)
Radix Albus Paeoniae Lactiflorae (*Bai Shao*)
prepared Radix Rehmanniae (*Shu Di*)
Radix Saussureae Seu Vladimiriae (*Mu Xiang*)

In case of fatigue with shortness of breath and a heavy, dragging feeling in the lower abdomen, add Radix Codonopsis Pilosulae (*Dang Shen*) and Radix Astragali Membranacei (*Huang Qi*). For incessant, clear vaginal discharge, add Semen Euryalis Ferocis (*Qian Shi*) and Fructus Rosae Laevigatae (*Jin Ying Zi*). In case of polyuria and nocturia, add Fructus Alpiniae Oxyphyllae (*Yi Zhi Ren*), Ootheca Mantidis (*Sang Piao Xiao*), and Os Draconis (*Long Gu*).

Unnamed formula given by the authors of *Concise Traditional Chinese Gynecology*

Radix Angelicae Sinensis (*Dang Gui*)
Semen Cuscutae (*Tu Si Zi*)
Cornu Degelatinum Cervi (*Lu Jiao Shuang*)
Radix Morindae Officinalis (*Ba Ji Tian*)
Sclerotium Poriae Cocoris (*Fu Ling*)

Unnamed formula given by Shang Xian-ming *et al.*

Herba Epimedii (*Xian Ling Pi*)
Radix Morindae Officinalis (*Ba Ji Tian*)
Semen Cuscutae (*Tu Si Zi*)
Fructus Rubi (*Fu Pen Zi*)
prepared Radix Rehmanniae (*Shu Di*)
Radix Angelicae Sinensis (*Dang Gui*)
Rhizoma Ligustici Wallichii (*Chuan Xiong*)
Radix Albus Paeoniae Lactiflorae (*Bai Shao*)
Placenta Hominis (*Zi He Che*)
Semen Leonuri Heterophylli (*Chong Wei Zi*)
Fructus Lycii Chinensis (*Gou Qi Zi*)
Fructus Schizandrae Chinensis (*Wu Wei Zi*)

This formula is similar to *Er Si Wu He Ji* given above.

Unnamed formula given by He Yuan-lin and Jiang Chang-yun, authors of *Fu Ke Bing Liang Fang (Fine Formulas for Gynecological Diseases)*

Radix Codonopsis Pilosulae (*Dang Shen*)
Rhizoma Atractylodis Macrocephalae (*Bai Zhu*)
Sclerotium Poriae Cocoris (*Fu Ling*)

Radix Albus Paeoniae Lactiflorae (*Bai Shao*)
Rhizoma Ligustici Wallichii (*Chuan Xiong*)
mix-fried Radix Glycyrrhizae (*Zhi Gan Cao*)
Radix Angelicae Sinensis (*Dang Gui*)
prepared Radix Rehmanniae (*Shu Di*)
Semen Cuscutae (*Tu Si Zi*)
Cortex Eucommiae Ulmoidis (*Du Zhong*)
Cornu Degelatinum Cervi (*Lu Jiao Shuang*)
Fructus Zanthoxyli Bungeani (*Chuan Jiao*)
Placenta Hominis (*Zi He Che*)
Radix Salviae Miltiorrhizae (*Dan Shen*)
Rhizoma Cyperi Rotundi (*Xiang Fu*)

Another unnamed formula from He and Jiang

Herba Cistanchis (*Rou Cong Rong*)
Fructus Rubi (*Fu Pen Zi*)
Semen Cnidii Monnieri (*She Chuang Zi*)
Rhizoma Ligustici Wallichii (*Chuan Xiong*)
Radix Angelicae Sinensis (*Dang Gui*)
Semen Cuscutae (*Tu Si Zi*)
Radix Albus Paeoniae Lactiflorae (*Bai Shao*)
Concha Ostreae (*Mu Li*)
Os Sepiae Seu Sepiellae (*Wu Zei Gu*)
Fructus Schizandrae Chinensis (*Wu Wei Zi*)
Radix Ledebouriellae Sesloidis (*Fang Feng*)
Radix Scutellariae Baicalensis (*Huang Qin*)
Folium Artemesiae Argyii (*Ai Ye*)

He and Jiang say that this formula is neither hot nor cold and that it assists yin to conceive. However, my interpretation of this formula is that it supplements kidney yang in order to generate *jing* essence without giving rise to evil heat.

Another unnamed formula from He and Jiang

Folium Artemesiae Argyii (*Ai Ye*)
Rhizoma Cyperi Rotundi (*Xiang Fu*)
Radix Angelicae Sinensis (*Dang Gui*)
Radix Dipsaci (*Xu Duan*)
Fructus Evodiae Rutecarpae (*Wu Zhu Yu*)
Rhizoma Ligustici Wallichii (*Chuan Xiong*)
Radix Albus Paeoniae Lactiflorae (*Bai Shao*)
Radix Astragali Membranacei (*Huang Qi*)
prepared Radix Rehmanniae (*Shu Di*)
Cortex Cinnamomi (*Rou Gui*)

He and Jiang say this formula is for a vacuity cold uterus with chilly pain in the lower abdomen and a delayed period with pale, scant blood, reduced sexual desire, low back and knee soreness and weakness, and a deep, weak or deep, choppy/astringent pulse.

Another unnamed formula from He and Jiang

Rhizoma Atractylodis Macrocephalae (*Bai Zhu*)
Radix Morindae Officinalis (*Ba Ji Tian*)
Radix Codonopsis Pilosulae (*Dang Shen*)
Cortex Eucommiae Ulmoidis (*Du Zhong*)
Semen Cuscutae (*Tu Si Zi*)
Radix Dioscoreae Oppositae (*Shan Yao*)
Semen Euryalis Ferocis (*Qian Shi*)
Cortex Cinnamomi (*Rou Gui*)
Radix Praeparatus Aconiti Carmichaeli (*Fu Pian*)
Fructus Psoraleae Corylifoliae (*Bu Gu Zhi*)

This formula is for more pronounced vacuity cold uterus.

Shen Shi Tang

prepared Radix Rehmanniae (*Shu Di*)
Radix Dioscoreae Oppositae (*Shan Yao*)
Rhizoma Atractylodis Macrocephalae (*Bai Zhu*)
Sclerotium Poriae Cocoris (*Fu Ling*)
Rhizoma Alismatis (*Ze Xie*)
Fructus Lycii Chinensis (*Gou Qi*)
Radix Morindae Officinalis (*Ba Ji Tian*)
Semen Cuscutae (*Tu Si Zi*)
Cortex Cinnamomi (*Rou Gui*)
Radix Praeparatus Aconiti Carmichaeli (*Fu Zi*)
Cornu Cervi (*Lu Jiao*)
Fructus Psoraleae Corylifoliae (*Bu Gu Zhi*)
Pericarpium Citri Reticulatae (*Chen Pi*)

This formula is based on *Jin Gui Shen Qi Wan* plus ingredients to nourish the essence and rectify the qi while keeping the prescription easily digestible.

Zan Yu Dan

Radix Praeparatus Aconiti Carmichaeli (*Fu Zi*)
Cortex Cinnamomi (*Rou Gui*)
Herba Cistanchis (*Rou Cong Rong*)
Radix Morindae Officinalis (*Ba Ji Tian*)
Herba Epimedii (*Xian Ling Pi*)
Rhizoma Curculiginis Orchoidis (*Xian Mao*)
Semen Cnidii Monnieri (*She Chuang Zi*)
Semen Allii Tuberosi (*Jiu Zi*)
Fructus Corni Officinalis (*Shan Zhu Yu*)
Cortex Eucommiae Ulmoidis (*Du Zhong*)
prepared Radix Rehmanniae (*Shu Di*)
Fructus Lycii Chinensis (*Gou Qi Zi*)
Rhizoma Atractylodis Macrocephalae (*Bai Zhu*)

Wen Shen Wan

prepared Radix Rehmanniae (*Shu Di*)
Fructus Corni Officinalis (*Zhu Rou*)
Radix Morindae Officinalis (*Ba Ji*)
Radix Angelicae Sinensis (*Dang Gui*)
Semen Cuscutae (*Tu Si Zi*)
Cornu Parvum Cervi (*Lu Rong*)
Fructus Alpiniae Oxyphyllae (*Yi Zhi Ren*)
Radix Rehmanniae (*Sheng Di*)
Cortex Eucommiae Ulmoidis (*Du Zhong*)
Sclerotium Pararadicis Poriae Cocoris (*Fu Shen*)
Radix Dioscoreae Oppositae (*Shan Yao*)
Radix Polygalae Tenuifoliae (*Yuan Zhi*)
Radix Dipsaci (*Xu Duan*)
Semen Cnidii Monnieri (*She Chuang Zi*)

Wu and Qi, authors of *Zhong Yi Fu Ke Zhi Liao Shou Ce (A Handbook of TCM Gynecological Treatment)*, say that, for predominant kidney yang vacuity, one can add Radix Morindae Officinalis (*Ba Ji Tian*), Rhizoma Curculiginis Orchoidis (*Xian Mao*), and Herba Epimedii (*Xian Ling Pi*) to warm the kidneys and strengthen yang. According to these authors, this formula can also be used for predominant kidney yin vacuity infertility by deleting Cornu Parvum Cervi (*Lu Rong*) and adding Plastrum Testudinis (*Gui Ban*), Radix Albus Paeoniae Lactiflorae (*Bai Shao*), and Cortex Radicis Lycii Chinensis (*Di Gu Pi*).

Jia Jian Wen Shen Wan

prepared Radix Rehmanniae (*Shu Di*)
Fructus Evodiae Rutecarpae (*Wu Zhu Yu*)
Radix Morindae Officinalis (*Ba Ji Tian*)
Radix Angelicae Sinensis (*Dang Gui*)
Semen Cuscutae (*Tu Si Zi*)

Cornum Parvum Cervi (*Lu Rong*)
Cortex Eucommiae Ulmoidis (*Du Zhong*)
Radix Dioscoreae Oppositae (*Shan Yao*)
Radix Dipsaci (*Xu Duan*)
Fructus Lycii Chinensis (*Gou Qi*)
Radix Astragali Membranacei (*Huang Qi*)
Semen Cnidii Monnieri (*She Chuang Zi*)

Er Xian Tang Jia Jian

Rhizoma Curculiginis Orchoidis (*Xian Mao*)
Herba Epimedii (*Xian Ling Pi*)
Radix Morindae Officinalis (*Ba Ji Tian*)
Radix Astragali Membranacei (*Huang Qi*)
scorched Rhizoma Atractylodis Macrocephalae (*Bai Zhu*)
Radix Angelicae Sinensis (*Dang Gui*)
prepared Radix Rehmanniae (*Shu Di*)
Fructus Corni Officinalis (*Shan Zhu Yu*)
Conchae Ostreae (*Mu Li*)

This formula is given by Guo Yuan, author of *Shi Yong Zhong Xi Yi Jie He Fu Chan Ke Zheng Zhi (Proven Treatments in Practical Integrated Chinese-Western Gynecology & Obstetrics)*. It is for the treatment of kidney/spleen yang vacuity.

Jin Lian Zhong Zi Fang

Radix Angelicae Sinensis (*Dang Gui*)
Cortex Cinnamomi (*Gui Xin*)
Dens Draconis (*Long Yan*)
Radix Linderae Strychnifoliae (*Wu Yao*)
Fructus Alpiniae Oxyphyllae (*Yi Zhi*)
Cortex Eucommiae Ulmoidis (*Du Zhong*)
Rhizoma Acori Graminei (*Chang Pu*)
Fructus Evodiae Rutecarpae (*Wu Zhu Yu*)

Sclerotium Pararadicis Poriae Cocoris (*Fu Shen*)
Radix Cyathulae (*Chuan Niu Xi*)
Radix Gentianae Macrophyllae (*Qin Jiao*)
Herba Cum Radice Asari Seiboldi (*Xi Xin*)
Radix Platycodi Grandiflori (*Jie Geng*)
Radix Ledebouriellae Sesloidis (*Fang Feng*)
Rhizoma Pinelliae Ternatae (*Ban Xia*)
Radix Albus Paeoniae Lactiflorae (*Bai Shao*)
dry Rhizoma Zingiberis (*Gan Jiang*)
Fructus Zanthoxyli Bungeani (*Chuan Jiao*)
Radix Praeparatus Aconiti Carmichaeli (*Fu Zi*)
Concha Ostreae (*Mu Li*)

This formula is given by Du Jie-hui for kidney/spleen yang vacuity with cold uterus (*gong han*). In this case, yang vacuity has led to a loss of normalcy in the transportation and transformation of body fluids. Being heavy, these have percolated down to the lower burner to obstruct the free flow of qi and blood. Some amount of fluid dampness has congealed into phlegm and there is actual cold causing stagnation beyond just a lack of yang qi to move the qi and blood freely.

Zhong Si Wan

Radix Praeparatus Aconiti Carmichaeli (*Fu Zi*)
Sclerotium Poriae Cocoris (*Bai Fu Ling*)
Radix Cynanchi (*Bai Wei*)
Rhizoma Pinelliae Ternatae (*Ban Xia*)
Cortex Eucommiae Ulmoidis (*Du Zhong*)
Cortex Cinnamomi (*Gui Xin*)
Cortex Magnoliae Officinalis (*Hou Po*)
Radix Gentianae Macrophyllae (*Qin Jiao*)
Radix Ledebouriellae Sesloidis (*Fang Feng*)
dry Rhizoma Zingiberis (*Gan Jiang*)
Radix Achyranthis Bidentatae (*Niu Xi*)

Radix Glehniae Littoralis (*Sha Shen*)
Herba Cum Radice Asari Seiboldi (*Xi Xin*)
Radix Panacis Ginseng (*Ren Shen*)

This formula, also given by Du Jie-hui, likewise treats a cold, damp uterus complicated by an element of phlegm due to kidney/spleen yang vacuity.

Wen Bao Yin

Rhizoma Atractylodis Macrocephalae (*Bai Zhu*)
Radix Morindae Officinalis (*Ba Ji*)
Radix Panacis Ginseng (*Ren Shen*)
Cortex Eucommiae Ulmoidis (*Du Zhong*)
Semen Cuscutae (*Tu Si Zi*)
Semen Euryalis Ferocis (*Qian Shi*)
Cortex Cinnamomi (*Rou Gui*)
Radix Praeparatus Aconiti Carmichaeli (*Fu Zi*)
Fructus Psoraleae Corylifoliae (*Bu Gu Zhi*)
Radix Dioscoreae Oppositae (*Shan Yao*)

This is Fu Qing-zhu's famous formula.

Wen Bao Yin Jia Wei

earth-fried Rhizoma Atractylodis Macrocephalae (*Bai Zhu*)
Ramulus Cinnamomi (*Gui Zhi*)
salt-fried Radix Morindae Officinalis (*Xi Ba Ji*)
Radix Codonopsis Pilosulae (*Dang Shen*)
stir-fried Cortex Eucommiae Ulmoidis (*Du Zhong*)
wine-fried Semen Cuscutae (*Tu Si Zi*)
stir-fried Radix Dioscoreae Oppositae (*Shan Yao*)
stir-fried Semen Euryalis Ferocis (*Qian Shi*)
Radix Praeparatus Aconiti Carmichaeli (*Fu Zi*)
salt-fried Fructus Psoraleae Corylifoliae (*Bu Gu Zhi*)

vinegar-fried Rhizoma Cyperi Rotundi (*Xiang Fu*)
stir-fried Fructus Foeniculi Vulgaris (*Hui Xiang*)
Herba Epimedii (*Xian Ling Pi*)
salt-washed Rhizoma Curculiginis Orchoidis (*Xian Mao*)
Radix Dipsaci (*Xu Duan*)

This formula is meant to supplement the kidneys and spleen and strengthen yang at the same time as filling and nourishing the extraordinary vessels.

Kuan Dai Tang

earth-fried Rhizoma Atractylodis Macrocephalae (*Bai Zhu*)
Radix Dioscoreae Oppositae (*Shan Yao*)
prepared Radix Rehmanniae (*Shu Di*)
wine-washed Radix Morindae Officinalis (*Ba Ji*)
salt-fried Fructus Psoraleae Corylifoliae (*Bu Gu Zhi*)
stir-fried Cortex Eucommiae Ulmoidis (*Du Zhong*)
Herba Cistanchis (*Rou Cong Rong*)
wine-fried Radix Albus Paeoniae Lactiflorae (*Bai Shao*)
stir-fried Fructus Schizandrae Chinensis (*Wu Wei*)
Semen Nelumbinis Nuciferae (*Lian Rou*)

This formula supplements the kidneys and spleen, scatters cold, restrains the *dai*, and consolidates the *chong* and *ren*. Cong Chun-yu indicates it for kidney/spleen yang vacuity with cold and dampness accumulating internally thus resulting in infertility.

Wen Gong Bu Xue Tang

Radix Codonopsis Pilosulae (*Dang Shen*)
Rhizoma Atractylodis Macrocephalae (*Bai Zhu*)
Sclerotium Poriae Cocoris (*Fu Ling*)
Radix Angelicae Sinensis (*Dang Gui*)
prepared Radix Rehmanniae (*Shu Di*)

Radix Polygoni Multiflori (*Shou Wu*)
Semen Cuscutae (*Tu Si Zi*)
Herba Epimedii (*Yin Yang Huo*)
Fluoritum (*Zi Shi Ying*)
Herba Leonuri Heterophylli (*Yi Mu Cao*)

This formula is given by Huang Shou-ren for the treatment of vacuity cold infertility due to yang insufficiency failing to warm the uterus and fill the essence. As Huang says, when the uterus does not receive nourishment, conception cannot take place. This formula nourishes liver blood as well as kidney yang and also does address a minor element of blood stasis.

Unnamed formula given by Wu and Qi in *Zhong Yi Fu Ke Zhi Liao Shou Ce (A Handbook of TCM Gynecological Treatment)*

Radix Angelicae Sinensis (*Dang Gui*)
Radix Morindae Officinalis (*Ba Ji Tian*)
Herba Epimedii (*Yin Yang Huo*)
Radix Dipsaci (*Chuan Duan*)
stir-fried Cortex Eucommiae Ulmoidis (*Du Zhong*)

Unnamed formula given by Liu and Liu

Radix Codonopsis Pilosulae (*Dang Shen*)
Rhizoma Atractylodis Macrocephalae (*Bai Zhu*)
Sclerotium Poriae Cocoris (*Fu Ling*)
mix-fried Radix Glycyrrhizae (*Zhi Gan Cao*)
Radix Angelicae Sinensis (*Dang Gui*)
Rhizoma Ligustici Wallichii (*Chuan Xiong*)
prepared Radix Rehmanniae (*Shu Di*)
Radix Albus Paeoniae Lactiflorae (*Bai Shao*)
Semen Cuscutae (*Tu Si Zi*)
Cortex Eucommiae Ulmoidis (*Du Zhong*)
Fructus Zanthoxyli Bungeani (*Chuan Jiao*)

Cornu Degelatinum Cervi (*Lu Jiao Shuang*)

Shen Yin Xu
Kidney Yin Vacuity

Pathognomonic manifestations: Chronic infertility or infertility in an older woman whose body tends to be thin, early menses, amount scant, color red with no clots, or normal menstruation, facial color yellow but red cheeks, low back and knee soreness and weakness, dizziness, blurred vision, both eyes dry and astringent, heart palpitations, loss of sleep, easily agitated emotionally, a dry mouth and red lips, vexatious heat in the five centers or hearts, possible heel pain, afternoon low grade or tidal fever, night sweats, a red, possibly dry tongue or red tongue tip with scant coating, and a thready, rapid or thready, wiry pulse

Therapeutic principles: Enrich yin and nourish the blood, balance the *chong* and boost the essence

Rx: *Yang Jing Zhong Yu Tang*

prepared Radix Rehmanniae (*Shu Di*)
Radix Angelicae Sinensis (*Dang Gui*)
Radix Albus Paeoniae Lactiflorae (*Bai Shao*)
Fructus Corni Officinalis (*Rou Zhu*)

This is another of Fu Qing-zhu's formulas. The authors of *Zhong Yi Fu Chan Ke Xue (A Study of TCM Gynecology & Obstetrics)* suggest adding Radix Dipsaci (*Xu Duan*), Ramus Loranthis Seu Visci (*Ji Sheng*), and Radix Polygoni Multiflori (*Shou Wu*).

Yang Jing Zhong Yu Tang Jia Nu Zhen Zi Han Lian Cao

Radix Angelicae Sinensis (*Dang Gui*)
Radix Albus Paeoniae Lactiflorae (*Bai Shao*)

prepared Radix Rehmanniae (*Shu Di*)
Fructus Corni Officinalis (*Shan Zhu Yu*)
Fructus Ligustri Lucidi (*Nu Zhen Zi*)
Herba Ecliptae Prostratae (*Han Lian Cao*)

If the body is emaciated or thin with heat in the five hearts and yin vacuity with effulgent fire, add Cortex Radicis Moutan (*Dan Pi*), Cortex Radicis Lycii (*Di Gu Pi*), Cortex Phellodendri (*Huang Bai*), and Plastrum Testudinis (*Gui Ban*).

Jia Wei Di Huang Tang

Radix Rehmanniae (*Sheng Di*)
prepared Radix Rehmanniae (*Shu Di*)
stir-fried Radix Dioscoreae Oppositae (*Shan Yao*)
Cortex Radicis Moutan (*Dan Pi*)
Fructus Corni Officinalis (*Shan Zhu Yu*)
Sclerotium Poriae Cocoris (*Fu Ling*)
Rhizoma Alismatis (*Ze Xie*)
Herba Ecliptae Prostratae (*Han Lian Cao*)
Fructus Ligustri Lucidi (*Nu Zhen Zi*)
Ramus Loranthis Seu Visci (*Sang Ji Sheng*)
Radix Dipsaci (*Xu Duan*)
stir-fried Radix Cyathulae (*Chuan Niu Xi*)

This formula might also be called *Liu Wei Di Huang Wan Jia Wei*. To that famous standard guiding formula for kidney yin vacuity it adds ingredients to further enrich the yin while at the same time ensuring the free flow of blood to and in the uterus.

Liu Wei Di Huang Tang Jia Jian

Radix Rehmanniae (*Sheng Di*)
Fructus Corni Officinalis (*Shan Zhu Yu*)
Radix Dioscoreae Oppositae (*Shan Yao*)

43

Cortex Radicis Moutan (*Dan Pi*)
Rhizoma Alismatis (*Ze Xie*)
Cortex Radicis Lycii Chinensis (*Di Gu Pi*)
Radix Angelicae Sinensis (*Dang Gui*)
Radix Albus Paeoniae Lactiflorae (*Bai Shao*)
Herba Ecliptae Prostratae (*Han Lian Cao*)
Fructus Ligustri Lucidi (*Nu Zhen Zi*)
Flos Carthami Tinctorii (*Hong Hua*)
Radix Dipsaci (*Xu Duan*)

If there is thirst and a dry tongue coating, add Radix Scrophulariae Ningpoensis (*Yuan Shen*), Rhizoma Anemarrhenae (*Zhi Mu*), and Tuber Ophiopogonis Japonicae (*Mai Dong*). If there is vexation and agitation and loss of sleep, add Semen Biotae Orientalis (*Bai Zi Ren*), Fructus Schizandrae Chinensis (*Wu Wei Zi*), and Semen Zizyphi Spinosae (*Suan Zao Ren*).

Yu Yin Tang Jia Jian

prepared Radix Rehmanniae (*Shu Di*)
Radix Dioscoreae Oppositae (*Shan Yao*)
Radix Dipsaci (*Chuan Duan*)
Ramus Loranthi Seu Visci (*Sang Ji Sheng*)
Radix Achyranthis Bidentatae (*Huai Niu Xi*)
Fructus Corni Officinalis (*Shan Zhu Yu*)
Radix Albus Paeoniae Lactiflorae (*Bai Shao*)
Concha Ostreae (*Mu Li*)
Cortex Eucommiae Ulmoidis (*Du Zhong*)
Os Sepiae Seu Sepiellae (*Hai Piao Xiao*)
Semen Cuscutae (*Tu Si Zi*)
Plastrum Testudinis (*Gui Ban*)

This formula by Han Bai-ling includes both heavy, yang repressing ingredients and astringing ingredients. The astringing ingredients (Concha Ostreae and Os Sepiae) are meant to consolidate the *chong* and stop any night sweats, but also help to control any tendency to early menstruation.

Unnamed formula from *Concise Traditional Chinese Gynecology*

Radix Angelicae Sinensis (*Dang Gui*)
Radix Albus Paeoniae Lactiflorae (*Bai Shao*)
prepared Radix Rehmanniae (*Shu Di*)
Fructus Corni Officinalis (*Shan Zhu Yu*)
Cortex Radicis Moutan (*Dan Pi*)

This is another of the typically truncated formulas from this book. Its ingredients are meant to nourish liver blood at the same time as enriching kidney yin and cooling the blood.

Zuo Gui Wan

prepared Radix Rehmanniae (*Shu Di*)
Radix Dioscoreae Oppositae (*Shan Yao*)
Fructus Lycii Chinensis (*Gou Qi Zi*)
Fructus Corni Officinalis (*Shan Zhu Yu*)
Semen Cuscutae (*Tu Si Zi*)
Radix Cyathulae (*Chuan Niu Xi*)
Gelatinum Cornu Cervi (*Lu Jiao Jiao*)
Gelatinum Plastri Testudinis (*Gui Ban Jiao*)

Shen Mi Zhong Zi Fang

Radix Angelicae Sinensis (*Dang Gui*)
Radix Rehmanniae (*Sheng Di*)
Radix Albus Paeoniae Lactiflorae (*Shao Yao*)
Radix Scutellariae Baicalensis (*Huang Qin*)
Cortex Radicis Moutan (*Dan Pi*)
Rhizoma Anemarrhenae (*Zhi Mu*)
Cortex Eucommiae Ulmoidis (*Du Zhong*)

Rhizoma Corydalis Yanhusuo (*Yuan Hu*)
Rhizoma Cyperi Rotundi (*Xiang Fu*)
Pericarpium Citri Reticulatae (*Chen Pi*)
Fructus Amomi (*Sha Ren*)
Fructus Schizandrae Chinensis (*Bei Wu Wei*)
Rhizoma Ligustici Wallichii (*Chuan Xiong*)
Medulla Junci Effusi (*Deng Cao*)
Herba Lophatheri Gracilis (*Dan Zhu Ye*)
Shi Zao Rou (石枣肉) stone date meat, presumably pitted Fructus
　　Zizyphi Jujubae

This formula nourishes yin and clears heat, rectifies the qi and
quickens the blood. Du Jie-hui says that it is not alright to add and
subtract from this prescription.

Ba Sheng Dan

Fructus Tribuli Terrestris (*Sha Ji Li*)
Radix Dipsaci (*Chuan Xu Duan*)
Fructus Rubi (*Fu Pen Zi*)
Fructus Lycii Chinensis (*Gou Qi Zi*)
Fructus Corni Officinalis (*Shan Zhu*)
Semen Cuscutae (*Tu Si Zi*)
Semen Euryalis Ferocis (*Qian Shi*)
Stamen Nelumbinis Nuciferae (*Lian Xu*)

Du Jie-hui says this formula supplements the liver and boosts the
kidneys in the treatment of kidney yin vacuity infertility.

Ji Kun Da Zao Wan

Placenta Hominis (*Zi He Che*)
Radix Angelicae Sinensis (*Dang Gui*)
Radix Panacis Ginseng (*Ren Shen*)
Radix Dioscoreae Oppositae (*Shan Yao*)

Cortex Eucommiae Ulmoidis (*Du Zhong*)
Tuber Asparagi Cochinensis (*Tian Dong*)
Tuber Ophiopogonis Japonicae (*Mai Dong*)
prepared Radix Rehmanniae (*Shu Di*)
Cortex Phellodendri (*Huang Bai*)

Du Jie-hui says that one can also add Fructus Schizandrae Chinensis (*Wu Wei Zi*). This formula supplements the kidneys and boosts the essence, boosts the qi and nourishes the blood in cases where kidney yin is insufficient and essence and blood are deficient and diminished.

Yu Qing Wan

Pericarpium Citri Reticulatae (*Chen Pi*)
Fructus Corni Officinalis (*Shan Zhu Yu*)
stir-fried Rhizoma Corydalis Yanhusuo (*Hu Suo*)
prepared Radix Rehmanniae (*Di Huang*)
Rhizoma Cyperi Rotundi (*Xiang Fu*)
Radix Angelicae Sinensis (*Dang Gui*)
Radix Scutellariae Baicalensis (*Tiao Qin*)
Rhizoma Atractylodis Macrocephalae (*Bai Zhu*)
Fructus Rubi (*Fu Pen Zi*)
Fructus Amomi (*Sha Ren*)
Rhizoma Ligustici Wallichii (*Chuan Xiong*)

This formula supplements the kidneys and transforms phlegm, rectifies the qi and regulates the menses. It is indicated for infertility due to kidney yin vacuity with simultaneous phlegm dampness and qi stagnation.

Qing Gu Zi Shen Tang Jia Wei

wine-washed Fructus Lycii Chinensis (*Gou Qi*)
Cortex Radicis Moutan (*Dan Pi*)
Radix Rehmanniae (*Sheng Di*)

Radix Scrophulariae Ningpoensis (*Yuan Shen*)
Radix Glehniae Littoralis (*Sha Shen*)
Fructus Schizandrae Chinensis (*Wu Wei Zi*)
Rhizoma Anemarrhenae (*Zhi Mu*)
salt-fried Cortex Phellodendri (*Huang Bai*)
Cortex Albizziae Julibrissinis (*He Huan Pi*)
vinegar-fried Rhizoma Cyperi Rotundi (*Xiang Fu*)
Concha Ostreae (*Mu Li*)
Semen Citri Reticulatae (*Ju He*)

This formula is based on one from *Fu Shan Nu Ke (Fu Shan's Gynecology)* as modified by Cong Chun-yu. Cong says to administer this prescription for infertility accompanied by thinness and early periods due to yin vacuity and blood heat complicated liver qi stagnation. Cong advises administering this formula before the period alternating with formula below after the period.

Liang Di Tang Jia Wei

Radix Scrophulariae Ningpoensis (*Yuan Shen*)
Radix Rehmanniae (*Sheng Di*)
Tuber Ophiopogonis Japonicae (*Mai Dong*)
Cortex Radicis Lycii (*Di Gu Pi*)
Radix Albus Paeoniae Lactiflorae (*Bai Shao*)
Gelatinum Corii Asini (*E Jiao*)
Radix Angelicae Sinensis (*Dang Gui*)
Pericarpium Citri Reticulatae (*Chen Pi*)

Qing Xue Yang Yin Tang

Radix Rehmanniae (*Sheng Di*)
Cortex Radicis Moutan (*Dan Pi*)
Radix Albus Paeoniae Lactiflorae (*Bai Shao*)
Cortex Phellodendri (*Huang Bai*)
Radix Scrophulariae Ningpoensis (*Yuan Shen*)

Fructus Ligustri Lucidi (*Nu Zhen Zi*)
Herba Ecliptae Prostratae (*Han Lian Cao*)

The authors of *Zhong Yi Fu Chan Ke Xue (A Study of TCM Gynecology & Obstetrics)* recommend this formula for the treatment yin vacuity with internal heat.

Yang Jing Zhong Yu Tang Jia Wei

prepared Radix Rehmanniae (*Shu Di*)
Radix Rehmanniae (*Sheng Di*)
wine-washed Radix Angelicae Sinensis (*Dang Gui*)
wine-washed Radix Albus Paeoniae Lactiflorae (*Bai Shao*)
stir-fried Fructus Corni Officinalis (*Shan Zhu*)
Fructus Schizandrae Chinensis (*Wu Wei Zi*)
Massa Medica Fermentata (*Shen Qu*)

Cong Chun-yu has added Radix Rehmanniae and Fructus Schizandrae to this formula to further supplement the kidneys and relax the liver.

Yang Jing Zhong Yu Tang Jia Jian

Fructus Rubi (*Fu Pen Zi*)
Fructus Lycii Chinensis (*Gou Qi Zi*)
stir-fried Radix Albus Paeoniae Lactiflorae (*Bai Shao*)
Radix Polygoni Multiflori (*Shou Wu*)
Rhizoma Polygonati (*Huang Jing*)
Herba Epimedii (*Xian Ling Pi*)
prepared Radix Rehmanniae (*Shu Di*)
Radix Rehmanniae (*Sheng Di*)
Herba Cynomorii Songarici (*Suo Yang*)
processed Plastrum Testudinis (*Gui Ban*)
Rhizoma Acori Graminei (*Chang Pu*)
Placenta Hominis (*Zi He Che*)
Tuber Ophiopogonis Japonicae (*Mai Dong*)

Unnamed formula given by Wu and Qi

Radix Angelicae Sinensis (*Dang Gui*)
Radix Albus Paeoniae Lactiflorae (*Bai Shao*)
prepared Radix Rehmanniae (*Shu Di*)
Fructus Corni Officinalis (*Shan Zhu*)
Radix Polygoni Multiflori (*Shou Wu*)
stir-fried Plastrum Testudinis (*Gui Ban*)
Fructus Ligustri Lucidi (*Nu Zhen Zi*)
Cornu Degelatinum Cervi (*Lu Jiao Shuang*)
stir-fried Cortex Eucommiae Ulmoidis (*Du Zhong*)

This formula treats kidney/liver dual vacuity where there is kidney yin vacuity, liver blood vacuity, and an element of yang vacuity as well.

Unnamed formula given by Liu and Liu

Cortex Radicis Lycii Chinensis (*Di Gu Pi*)
Cortex Radicis Moutan (*Dan Pi*)
Radix Glehniae Littoralis (*Sha Shen*)
Tuber Ophiopogonis Japonicae (*Mai Dong*)
Radix Scrophulariae Ningpoensis (*Yuan Shen*)
Fructus Schizandrae Chinensis (*Wu Wei Zi*)
Rhizoma Atractylodis Macrocephalae (*Bai Zhu*)
Herba Dendrobii (*Shi Hu*)

Unnamed formula given by He and Jiang

prepared Radix Rehmanniae (*Shu Di*)
Fructus Corni Officinalis (*Shan Zhu Yu*)
Radix Angelicae Sinensis (*Dang Gui*)
Radix Albus Paeoniae Lactiflorae (*Bai Shao*)
Placenta Hominis (*Zi He Che*)

He and Jiang say this formula is for insufficiency of blood and *jing* and amenorrhea or delayed periods with bodily weakness, a sallow yellow facial complexion, dizziness and tinnitus.

Another unnamed formula from He and Jiang

Cortex Radicis Moutan (*Dan Pi*)
Plastrum Testudinis (*Gui Ban*)
Fructus Ligustri Lucidi (*Nu Zhen Zi*)
Fructus Lycii Chinensis (*Gou Qi*)
prepared Radix Rehmanniae (*Shu Di*)
Fructus Corni Officinalis (*Shan Zhu Yu*)
Radix Angelicae Sinensis (*Dang Gui*)
Radix Albus Paeoniae Lactiflorae (*Bai Shao*)
Placenta Hominis (*Zi He Che*)

He and Jiang recommend this formula for blood and *jing* vacuity with bodily emaciation and vexatious heat in the five hearts.

Another unnamed formula from He and Jiang

prepared Radix Rehmanniae (*Shu Di*)
Fructus Corni Officinalis (*Shan Zhu Yu*)
Radix Dioscoreae Oppositae (*Shan Yao*)
Cortex Radicis Moutan (*Dan Pi*)
Sclerotium Poriae Cocoris (*Fu Ling*)
Rhizoma Alismatis (*Ze Xie*)
Rhizoma Cyperi Rotundi (*Xiang Fu*)

This formula is for kidney vacuity infertility with menstrual irregularity.

Yet another unnamed formula from He and Jiang

Tuber Asparagi Cochinensis (*Tian Dong*)

Tuber Ophiopogonis Japonicae (*Mai Dong*)
Rhizoma Acori Graminei (*Shi Chang Pu*)
Sclerotium Poriae Cocoris (*Fu Ling*)
Radix Codonopsis Pilosulae (*Dang Shen*)
Fructus Alpiniae Oxyphyllae (*Yi Zhi Ren*)
Fructus Lycii Chinensis (*Gou Qi Zi*)
Cortex Radicis Lycii Chinensis (*Di Gu Pi*)
Radix Polygalae Tenuifoliae (*Yuan Zhi*)

This formula treats an emaciated, weak women with too little blood to enable conception.

Wu Zi Tang

Fructus Rubi (*Fu Pen Zi*)
Semen Cuscutae (*Tu Si Zi*)
Fructus Ligustri Lucidi (*Nu Zhen Zi*)
Fructus Lycii Chinensis (*Gou Qi Zi*)
Fructus Rosae Laevigatae (*Jin Ying Zi*)
Radix Pseudostellariae (*Tai Zi Shen*)
Radix Rehmanniae (*Sheng Di*)
Rhizoma Polygonati (*Huang Jing*)
Fructus Corni Officinalis (*Shan Zhu Yu*)
Herba Cistanchis (*Rou Cong Rong*)
Radix Angelicae Sinensis (*Dang Gui*)
processed Radix Polygoni Multiflori (*Shou Wu*)

Dan Zhi Xiao Yao San Jia Gu Jing Wan

Cortex Radicis Moutan (*Dan Pi*)
Fructus Gardeniae Jasminoidis (*Zhi Zi*)
Radix Bupleuri (*Chai Hu*)
Radix Angelicae Sinensis (*Dang Gui*)
Radix Albus Paeoniae Lactiflorae (*Bai Shao*)
Rhizoma Atractylodis Macrocephalae (*Bai Zhu*)

Sclerotium Poriae Cocoris (*Fu Ling*)
Plastrum Testudinis (*Gui Ban*)
Radix Scutellariae Baicalensis (*Huang Qin*)
Cortex Phellodendri (*Huang Bai*)
Cortex Cedrelae (*Chun Gen Pi*)
Rhizoma Cyperi Rotundi (*Xiang Fu*)

Huang Shou-ren recommends modifying this basic combination with additions and subtractions for the treatment of vacuity heat infertility. It is an interesting approach since it does recognize that liver stagnation and depressive heat eventually injure and waste yin fluids. *In toto*, this formula addresses liver stagnation, depressive heat, damp heat or yin fire below, spleen vacuity and dampness, vacuity heat/heat in the blood *fen*, and yin and blood vacuity. Although Huang refers to this as a vacuity heat pattern, it is more complicated than those words would at first suggest.

Interestingly, Huang Shou-ren says that female infertility, in general, can be divided into vacuity cold, vacuity heat, and stasis and stagnation types. Once one understands the ramifications of all of these mechanisms and patterns, that seemingly simple statement becomes much more complex. Yet at the same time, that simple statement helps reduce that complexity down to three core issues. In other words, such seemingly simple statements are both deceptively simple and bearers of great brilliance deserving long thought and meditation.

Xue Xu
Blood Vacuity

Pathognomonic manifestations: Infertility, facial color sallow yellow, menses delayed, amount scant, color pale, dizziness, blurred vision, dry skin, heart palpitations, loss of sleep, constipation, stools closed and bound, insidious pain in the lower abdomen after menstruation, a pale, possibly dry tongue, and a thready, weak or vacuous, weak pulse

Therapeutic principles: Supplement the blood and boost the qi

Rx: *Ren Shen Yang Rong Tang*

Radix Panacis Ginseng (*Ren Shen*)
prepared Radix Rehmanniae (*Shu Di*)
Rhizoma Atractylodis Macrocephalae (*Bai Zhu*)
Radix Angelicae Sinensis (*Dang Gui*)
Radix Albus Paeoniae Lactiflorae (*Bai Shao*)
Sclerotium Poriae Cocoris (*Fu Ling*)
Radix Astragali Seu Hedysari (*Huang Qi*)
Cortex Cinnamomi (*Rou Gui*)
Fructus Schizandrae Chinensis (*Wu Wei Zi*)
Radix Polygalae Tenuifoliae (*Yuan Zhi*)
Pericarpium Citri Reticulatae (*Chen Pi*)
mix-fried Radix Glycyrrhizae (*Zhi Gan Cao*)
fresh Rhizoma Zingiberis (*Sheng Jiang*)
Fructus Zizyphi Jujubae (*Da Zao*)

Yang Jing Zhong Yu Tang

prepared Radix Rehmanniae (*Shu Di*)
stir-fried Radix Angelicae Sinensis (*Dang Gui*)
wine-fried Radix Albus Paeoniae Lactiflorae (*Bai Shao*)
Fructus Corni Officinalis (*Shan Zhu Yu*)

If blood vacuity is severe, add Cornu Cervi (*Lu Jiao Pian*) and Placenta Hominis (*Zi He Che*). Wu and Qi suggest adding prepared Radix Polygoni Multiflori (*Shou Wu*), Caulis Milletiae Seu Spatholobi (*Ji Xue Teng*), Fluoritum (*Zi Shi Ying*), and Herba Leonuri Heterophylli (*Yi Mu Cao*). Liu and Liu suggest adding Radix Codonopsis

Pilosulae (*Dang Shen*), Radix Astragali Membranacei (*Huang Qi*), and processed Radix Polygoni Multiflori (*Shou Wu*).

Unnamed formula given by Wu and Qi

Radix Angelicae Sinensis (*Dang Gui*)
Radix Albus Paeoniae Lactiflorae (*Bai Shao*)
prepared Radix Rehmanniae (*Shu Di*)
Radix Astragali Membranacei (*Huang Qi*)
Radix Dioscoreae Oppositae (*Shan Yao*)
Sclerotium Poriae Cocoris (*Bai Fu Ling*)
Radix Achyranthis Bidentatae (*Niu Xi*)
Herba Leonuri Heterophylli (*Yi Mu Cao*)
mix-fried Radix Glycyrrhizae (*Zhi Gan Cao*)

Yu Yin Bu Xue Tang

prepared Radix Rehmanniae (*Shu Di*)
Radix Dioscoreae Oppositae (*Shan Yao*)
Radix Angelicae Sinensis (*Dang Gui*)
Radix Albus Paeoniae Lactiflorae (*Bai Shao*)
Fructus Lycii Chinensis (*Gou Qi Zi*)
mix-fried Radix Glycyrrhizae (*Zhi Cao*)
Fructus Corni Officinalis (*Shan Zhu Yu*)
Cortex Radicis Moutan (*Dan Pi*)
Plastrum Testudinis (*Gui Ban*)
Carapax Amydae (*Bie Jia*)

This formula is similar to ones for the treatment of yin vacuity. It is given by Han Bai-ling who includes a discussion of kidney yin deficiency damage and blood vacuity. Under the signs and symptoms of blood vacuity, he lists heat in the hands, feet, and heart and for the therapeutic principles he gives supplement the blood and enrich yin.

Ba Zhen Yi Mu Wan

Radix Panacis Ginseng (*Ren Shen*)
stir-fried Rhizoma Atractylodis Macrocephalae (*Bai Zhu*)
Sclerotium Poriae Cocoris (*Fu Ling*)
Rhizoma Ligustici Wallichii (*Chuan Xiong*)
Radix Angelicae Sinensis (*Dang Gui*)
prepared Radix Rehmanniae (*Shu Di*)
mix-fried Radix Glycyrrhizae (*Zhi Gan Cao*)
vinegar-fried Radix Albus Paeoniae Lactiflorae (*Bai Shao*)
Herba Leonuri Heterophylli (*Yi Mu Cao*)

Bensky and Barolet give this formula for the treatment of infertility due to qi and blood vacuity complicated by an element of blood stasis.

Yu Lin Zhu Jia Jian

Radix Codonopsis Pilosulae (*Dang Shen*)
Radix Astragali Membranacei (*Huang Qi*)
stir-fried Rhizoma Atractylodis Macrocephalae (*Bai Zhu*)
Sclerotium Poriae Cocoris (*Fu Ling*)
Radix Angelicae Sinensis (*Dang Gui*)
Rhizoma Ligustici Wallichii (*Chuan Xiong*)
prepared Radix Rehmanniae (*Shu Di*)
Radix Albus Paeoniae Lactiflorae (*Bai Shao*)
Gelatinum Corii Asini (*E Jiao*)
Semen Cuscutae (*Tu Si Zi*)
Fructus Zanthoxyli Bungeani (*Chuan Jiao*)
Herba Epimedii (*Xian Ling Pi*)

In case of abnormal vaginal discharge whose amount is scant, reduced sexual desire, and a dry, astringent vagina, add Placenta Hominis (*Zi He Che*) and Cornu Degelatinum Cervi (*Lu Jiao Shuang*). For lower abdominal urgency and pain during menstruation, add Caulis Milletiae

Seu Spatholobi (*Ji Xue Teng*) and Herba Leonuri Heterophylli (*Yi Mu Cao*).

Dang Gui Shao Yao San

Radix Angelicae Sinensis (*Dang Gui*)
Radix Albus Paeoniae Lactiflorae (*Shao Yao*)
Sclerotium Poriae Cocoris (*Fu Ling*)
Rhizoma Atractylodis Macrocephalae (*Bai Zhu*)
Rhizoma Alismatis (*Ze Xie*)
Rhizoma Ligustici Wallichii (*Chuan Xiong*)

This formula is given for vacuity pattern infertility by Hong-yen Hsu. Bensky and Barolet explain this formula as treating disharmony between the liver and spleen. Liver blood is vacuous and this leads to qi stagnation. At the same time, the spleen's command of transportation and transformation of water has lost its normalcy and there is some element of qi vacuity and dampness.

Tiao Jing Zhong Zi Fang

Radix Angelicae Sinensis (*Dang Gui*)
prepared Radix Rehmanniae (*Shu Di*)
Rhizoma Cyperi Rotundi (*Xiang Fu*)
wine-fried Radix Albus Paeoniae Lactiflorae (*Bai Shao*)
Pericarpium Citri Reticulatae (*Chen Pi*)
Folium Artemesiae Argyii (*Ai Rong*)
Sclerotium Poriae Cocoris (*Fu Ling*)
mix-fried Radix Glycyrrhizae (*Zhi Cao*)
wine-fried Rhizoma Corydalis Yanhusuo (*Yuan Hu*)
Cortex Radicis Moutan (*Dan Pi*)
Fructus Corni Officinalis (*Shan Zhu Yu*)
blast-fried dry Rhizoma Zingiberis (*Gan Jiang*)
Rhizoma Ligustici Wallichii (*Chuan Xiong*)
Cortex Cinnamomi (*Guang Gui*)

fresh Rhizoma Zingiberis (*Sheng Jiang*)
Fructus Zizyphi Jujubae (*Da Hong Zao*)

Du Jie-hui recommends this formula for the treatment of infertility
due to blood vacuity and a cold uterus. Zhang Jian-xiu, author of
*Zhong Yi Zhi Liao Fu Ke Bing (The TCM Treatment of Gynecological
Diseases)*, calls a somewhat simplified version of this formula *Tiao
Jing Zhong Zi Tang*. In Zhang's version, Folium Artemesiae Argyii,
mix-fried Radix Glycyrrhizae, Rhizoma Desiccata Zingeberis, Cortex
Cinnamomi, and Fructus Zizyphi Jujubae are absent. Zhang says this
formula is for the treatment of liver/kidney insufficiency with liver
depression, qi stagnation and phlegm dampness obstruction and
stagnation. If the menses is early and the color of the blood is
purplish, Zhang recommends adding Radix Scutellariae Baicalensis
(*Huang Qin*). If the menses is late and its color is pale, then Zhang
says to add Cortex Cinnamomi (*Guan Gui*), dry Rhizoma Zingiberis
(*Gan Jiang*), and prepared Folium Artemesiae Argyii (*Ai*).

Dang Gui Yang Xue Tang Jia Wei

Radix Astragali Membranacei (*Huang Qi*)
Radix Angelicae Sinensis (*Dang Gui*)
Radix Polygoni Multiflori (*He Shou Wu*)
prepared Radix Rehmanniae (*Shu Di*)
stir-fried Rhizoma Atractylodis Macrocephalae (*Bai Zhu*)
Pericarpium Citri Reticulatae (*Chen Pi*)
Radix Glycyrrhizae (*Gan Cao*)

Gan Yu Qi Zhi
Liver Depression, Qi Stagnation

Pathognomonic manifestations: Menses early, late, at no fixed
schedule, amount scant, color dark red with small blood clots, lower
abdominal distention and pain when the period does come, premenstrual breast and flank distention and pain, emotional depression,

vexation and agitation, easily angered, belching, sighing, a cyan, dark facial color, a normal or dark red tongue with thin, white or yellow coating, and a wiry, slippery, forceful pulse

Therapeutic principles: Course the liver and resolve depression, nourish the blood and rectify the spleen

Rx: *Jia Wei Xiao Yao San*

Radix Bupleuri (*Chai Hu*)
Radix Albus Paeoniae Lactiflorae (*Bai Shao*)
Radix Angelicae Sinensis (*Dang Gui*)
Rhizoma Atractylodis Macrocephalae (*Bai Zhu*)
Rhizoma Cyperi Rotundi (*Xiang Fu*)
Herba Leonuri Heterophylli (*Yi Mu Cao*)
Cortex Albizziae Julibrissinis (*He Huan Pi*)
Flos Rosae Rugosae (*Mei Gui Hua*)
Tuber Curcumae (*Yu Jin*)
Caulis Polygoni Multiflori (*Ye Jiao Teng*)
Pericarpium Viridis Citri Reticulatae (*Qing Pi*)
Sclerotium Poriae Cocoris (*Fu Ling*)

Tiao Gan Li Qi Tang a.k.a. *Bai Ling Tiao Gan Tang*

Radix Angelicae Sinensis (*Dang Gui*)
Radix Albus Paeoniae Lactiflorae (*Bai Shao*)
Radix Bupleuri (*Chai Hu*)
Sclerotium Poriae Cocoris (*Fu Ling*)
Rhizoma Atractylodis Macrocephalae (*Bai Zhu*)
Cortex Radicis Moutan (*Dan Pi*)
Rhizoma Cyperi Rotundi (*Xiang Fu*)
Fructus Trichosanthis Kirlowii (*Gua Lou*)
Radix Achyranthis Bidentatae (*Huai Niu Xi*)
Fructus Meliae Toosendanis (*Chuan Lian*)
Semen Vaccariae Segetalis (*Wang Bu Liu Xing*)

Medulla Tetrapanacis Papyriferi (*Tong Cao*)
Radix Glycyrrhizae (*Gan Cao*)

This is Han Bai-ling's formula. If qi stagnation becomes more blood stasis and the breast distention is pronounced, Han deletes Radix Bupleuri and adds Rhizoma Ligustici Wallichii (*Chuan Xiong*), Radix Salviae Miltiorrhizae (*Dan Shen*) and Spina Gleditschiae (*Jiao Ci*) and may substitute Radix Rubrus Paeoniae Lactiflorae (*Chi Shao*) for Radix Albus Paeoniae Lactiflorae. In addition, if there is no spleen vacuity, Han deletes the Rhizoma Atractylodis Macrocephalae and Sclerotium Poriae Cocoris.

Chai Hu Shu Gan San

Radix Bupleuri (*Chai Hu*)
Pericarpium Citri Reticulatae (*Chen Pi*)
Radix Albus Paeoniae Lactiflorae (*Bai Shao*)
Fructus Citri Seu Ponciri (*Zhi Ke*)
mix-fried Radix Glycyrrhizae (*Zhi Gan Cao*)
Rhizoma Ligustici Wallichii (*Chuan Xiong*)
Rhizoma Cyperi Rotundi (*Xiang Fu*)

If there is breast distention and pain, add Caulis Akebiae Mutong (*Mu Tong*) and Tuber Curcumae (*Yu Jin*). If there are palpable lumps in the breast, add Semen Citri Reticulatae (*Ju He*), Fructus Liquidambaris Taiwaniae (*Lu Lu Tong*), and Squama Manitis (*Chuan Shan Jia*). If there is heat, add Cortex Radicis Moutan (*Dan Pi*) and Fructus Gardeniae Jasminoidis (*Zhi Zi*).

Jia Jian Chai Hu Shu Gan San

Radix Bupleuri (*Chai Hu*)
Fructus Citri Seu Ponciri (*Zhi Ke*)
Rhizoma Cyperi Rotundi (*Xiang Fu*)
Rhizoma Ligustici Wallichii (*Chuan Xiong*)

Fructus Liquidambaris Taiwaniae (*Lu Lu Tong*)
Radix Glycyrrhizae (*Gan Cao*)
Radix Albus Paeoniae Lactiflorae (*Bai Shao*)
Pericarpium Viridis Citri Reticulatae (*Qing Pi*)
Radix Salviae Miltiorrhizae (*Dan Shen*)

Wang and Wang say that, if there is breast pain, to add Semen Vaccariae Segetalis (*Wang Bu Liu Xing*), Semen Citri (*Ju He*), Retinervus Luffae (*Si Gua Luo*), and Fructus Meliae Toosendanis (*Jin Ling*). For simultaneous heat, add Cortex Radicis Moutan (*Dan Pi*) and Radix Scutellariae Baicalensis (*Huang Qin*). For simultaneous cold, add Ramulus Cinnamomi (*Gui Zhi*) and blast-fried Rhizoma Zingiberis (*Pao Jiang*). And for simultaneous blood stasis, add Semen Pruni Persicae (*Tao Ren*), Flos Carthami Tinctorii (*Hong Hua*), Feces Trogopterori Seu Pteromi (*Wu Ling Zhi*), and Pollen Typhae (*Pu Huang*).

Kai Yu Zhong Yu Tang

wine-fried Radix Albus Paeoniae Lactiflorae (*Bai Shao*)
wine-fried Rhizoma Cyperi Rotundi (*Xiang Fu*)
wine-fried Radix Angelicae Sinensis (*Dang Gui*)
earth-fried Rhizoma Atractylodis Macrocephalae (*Bia Zhu*)
wine-fried Cortex Radicis Moutan (*Dan Pi*)
Sclerotium Poriae Cocoris (*Fu Ling*)
Radix Trichosanthis Kirlowii (*Hua Fen*)

This formula is also known as *Jie Yu Zhong Yu Tang* and is from *Fu Qing Zhu Nu Ke (Fu Qing-zhu's Gynecology)*. Liu Lan-fang and Liu Dian-gong, authors of *Fu Ke San Bai Zheng (Three Hundred Gynecological Conditions)*, recommend the following modifications. For chest and lateral costal distention and fullness, delete Rhizoma Atractylodis Macrocephalae and add Pericarpium Viridis Citri Reticulatae (*Qing Pi*). For excessive dreams, loss of sleep, and lack of calm, add Semen Zizyphi Spinosae (*Zao Ren*). For breast distention and pain accompanied by a feeling of scorching heat or pain when touched, add Fructus Meliae Toosendanis (*Chuan Lian Zi*) and Herba Cum Radice Taraxaci Mongolici (*Pu Gong Ying*).

Unnamed formula given by Wu and Qi

Radix Bupleuri (*Chai Hu*)
Radix Angelicae Sinensis (*Dang Gui*)
Radix Albus Paeoniae Lactiflorae (*Bai Shao*)
Rhizoma Cyperi Rotundi (*Xiang Fu*)
Pericarpium Viridis Citri Reticulatae (*Qing Pi*)
Semen Cuscutae (*Tu Si Zi*)
stir-fried Cortex Eucommiae Ulmoidis (*Du Zhong*)
Caulis Milletiae Seu Spatholobi (*Ji Xue Teng*)
Fructus Corni Officinalis (*Shan Zhu*)
mix-fried Radix Glycyrrhizae (*Zhi Gan Cao*)

De Sheng Tang Jia Wei

Radix Angelicae Sinensis (*Dang Gui*)
Radix Albus Paeoniae Lactiflorae (*Bai Shao*)
Rhizoma Ligustici Wallichii (*Chuan Xiong*)
Herba Leonuri Heterophylli (*Yi Mu Cao*)
Radix Bupleuri (*Chai Hu*)
Radix Saussureae Seu Vladimiriae (*Guang Mu Xiang*)
Radix Salviae Miltiorrhizae (*Dan Shen*)
Fructus Meliae Toosendanis (*Chuan Lian Zi*)

Unnamed formula from *Concise Traditional Chinese Gynecology*

Radix Angelicae Sinensis (*Dang Gui*)
Radix Albus Paeoniae Lactiflorae (*Bai Shao*)
Sclerotium Poriae Cocoris (*Fu Ling*)
processed Rhizoma Cyperi Rotundi (*Xiang Fu*)
Tuber Curcumae (*Yu Jin*)

Unnamed formula given by Shang Xian-ming *et al.*

Radix Bupleuri (*Chai Hu*)
Rhizoma Cyperi Rotundi (*Xiang Fu*)
Cortex Albizziae Julibrissinis (*He Huan Pi*)
Semen Aesculi (*Suo Lou Zi*)
Radix Angelicae Sinensis (*Dang Gui*)
Rhizoma Ligustici Wallichii (*Chuan Xiong*)
Radix Albus Paeoniae Lactiflorae (*Bai Shao*)
prepared Radix Rehmanniae (*Shu Di*)
Radix Salviae Miltiorrhizae (*Dan Shen*)
Flos Rosae Rugosae (*Mei Gui Hua*)
Folium Citri Reticulatae (*Ju Ye*)
Semen Citri Reticulatae (*Ju He*)

Unnamed formula given by He and Jiang

Rhizoma Cyperi Rotundi (*Xiang Fu*)
Cortex Eucommiae Ulmoidis (*Du Zhong*)
Rhizoma Ligustici Wallichii (*Chuan Xiong*)
Radix Albus Paeoniae Lactiflorae (*Bai Shao*)
Radix Angelicae Sinensis (*Dang Gui*)
prepared Radix Rehmanniae (*Shu Di*)
Pericarpium Citri Reticulatae (*Chen Pi*)
Fructus Foeniculi Vulgaris (*Xia Hui*)
Rhizoma Corydalis Yanhusuo (*Yan Hu Suo*)
Herba Cistanchis (*Rou Cong Rong*)
Pericarpium Viridis Citri Reticulatae (*Qing Pi*)
Radix Linderae Strychnifoliae (*Wu Yao*)
Radix Scutellariae Baicalensis (*Huang Qin*)
Os Sepiae Seu Sepiellae (*Wu Zei Gu*)

This formula rectifies the qi and nourishes the blood, regulates the menses and promotes fertility.

Another unnamed formula from He and Jiang

Radix Angelicae Sinensis (*Dang Gui*)
Radix Albus Paeoniae Lactiflorae (*Bai Shao*)
Sclerotium Poriae Cocoris (*Fu Ling*)
Cortex Radicis Moutan (*Dan Pi*)
Rhizoma Cyperi Rotundi (*Xiang Fu*)
Radix Trichosanthis Kirlowii (*Hua Fen*)

This formula treats liver qi depression in older women with infertility whose periods come early, late, or at no fixed intervals. When the period comes, there is abdominal pain and it does not come easily. The blood is scant in amount and dark colored. There are small blood clots and before the period there is breast distention and pain with emotional depression, vexation and agitation, and easy anger. If chest and flank distention and fullness are severe, delete Rhizoma Atractylodis Macrocephalae and add Pericarpium Viridis Citri Reticulatae (*Qing Pi*) and Flos Immaturus Sophorae Japonicae (*Huai Hua*). If there is insomnia with many dreams, add Semen Zizyphi Spinosae (*Zao Ren*) and Caulis Polygoni Multiflori (*Ye Jiao Teng*). If there are lumps in the breasts, add Semen Vaccariae Segetalis (*Wang Bu Liu Xing*), Folium Citri (*Ju Ye*), Semen Citri (*Ju He*), and Fructus Liquidambaris Taiwaniae (*Lu Tong*). If there is breast distention and pain with a feeling of scorching heat and pain on pressure, add Fructus Meliae Toosendanis (*Chuan Lian Zi*) and Herba Cum Radicie Taraxaci Mongolici (*Pu Gong Ying*).

Yet another unnamed formula from He and Jiang

Cortex Radicis Lycii Chinensis (*Di Gu Pi*)
Cortex Radicis Moutan (*Dan Pi*)
Tuber Ophiopogonis Japonicae (*Mai Dong*)
Radix Scrophulariae Ningpoensis (*Yuan Shen*)
Radix Glehniae Littoralis (*Sha Shen*)
Rhizoma Atractylodis Macrocephalae (*Bai Zhu*)

Herba Dendrobii (*Shi Hu*)
Fructus Schizandrae Chinensis (*Wu Wei Zi*)

This formula is almost identical to one given above under yin vacuity. He and Jiang recommend this formula for depressive heat with chest and lateral costal distention and fullness, dizziness and tinnitus, and early or late period which comes at no fixed time, which is scant in amount and colored red, and a fine, rapid pulse. This underscores the fact that depressive heat can exhaust and damage yin fluids and easily give rise to yin vacuity while transforming into vacuity heat.

Shu Yu Tiao Jing Tang

Radix Bupleuri (*Chai Hu*)
Tuber Curcumae (*Yu Jin*)
Fructus Meliae Toosendanis (*Chuan Lian Zi*)
Rhizoma Cyperi Rotundi (*Xiang Fu*)
Radix Angelicae Sinensis (*Dang Gui*)
Rhizoma Ligustici Wallichii (*Chuan Xiong*)
Radix Albus Paeoniae Lactiflorae (*Bai Shao*)
Radix Rehmanniae (*Sheng Di*)
Fructus Mori Albi (*Sang Shen Zi*)
Fructus Citri Seu Ponciri (*Zhi Ke*)
Herba Leonuri Heterophylli (*Yi Mu Cao*)

For premenstrual breast distention and pain with lumps, add Spica Prunellae Vulgaris (*Xia Gu Cao*), Semen Citri (*Ju He*), Fructus Liquidambaris Taiwaniae (*Lu Lu Tong*), and Concha Ostreae (*Sheng Mu Li*). If the menses is scant and has difficulty being precipitated and abdominal pain is severe, add Rhizoma Curcumae Zedoariae (*E Zhu*), Rhizoma Corydalis Yanhusuo (*Yan Hu Suo*), and Pollen Typhae (*Sheng Pu Huang*) and delete Radix Rehmanniae and Fructus Mori Albi. If the tongue is red with a yellow coating and the pulse is wiry and rapid, add Cortex Radicis Moutan (*Dan Pi*), Fructus Gardeniae

Jasminoidis (*Zhi Zi*), and Radix Scrophulariae Ningpoensis (*Xuan Shen*) and delete Fructus Mori Albi.

Shao Fu Zhu Yu Tang Jia Jian

Radix Angelicae Sinensis (*Dang Gui*)
Rhizoma Ligustici Wallichii (*Chuan Xiong*)
Radix Rubrus Paeoniae Lactiflorae (*Chi Shao*)
Fructus Foeniculi Vulgaris (*Hui Xiang*)
Rhizoma Corydalis Yanhusuo (*Yan Hu Suo*)
Feces Trogopterori Seu Pteromi (*Wu Ling Zhi*)
Myrrha (*Mo Yao*)
Pollen Typhae (*Pu Huang*)
Rhizoma Cyperi Rotundi (*Xiang Fu*)
Radix Salviae Miltiorrhizae (*Dan Shen*)
Ramulus Cinnamomi (*Gui Zhi*)

This formula may be used if qi stagnation is complicated by blood stasis. If there is breast distention and pain with scorching heat, add Fructus Meliae Toosendanis (*Chuan Lian Zi*) and Herba Cum Radice Taraxaci Mongolici (*Pu Gong Ying*). If there are breast lumps and distention, add Semen Vaccariae Segetalis (*Wang Bu Liu Xing*), Folium Citri Reticulatae (*Ju Ye*), Semen Citri Reticulatae (*Ju He*), and Fructus Liquidambaris Taiwaniae (*Lu Lu Tong*). If there is chest and flank distention and fullness, add Pericarpium Viridis Citri Reticulatae (*Qing Pi*) and Flos Rosae Rugosae (*Mei Gui Hua*). If there are excessive dreams and sleep is not peaceful, add stir-fried Fructus Zizyphi Spinosae (*Zao Ren*) and Caulis Polygoni Multiflori (*Ye Jiao Teng*).

Unnamed formula given by Zhu Xiao-nan[1]

Rhizoma Cyperi Rotundi (*Xiang Fu*)
Cortex Albizziae Julibrissinis (*He Huan Pi*)
Fructus Perillae Frutescentis (*Su Zi*)
Fructus Liquidambaris (*Lu Lu Tong*)
Tuber Curcumae (*Yu Jin*)
stir-fried Rhizoma Atractylodis Macrocephalae (*Bai Zhu*)
stir-fried Radix Linderae Strychnifoliae (*Wu Yao*)
Pericarpium Citri Reticulatae (*Chen Pi*)
Fructus Immaturus Citri Seu Ponciri (*Zhi Shi*)

If there is breast distention, add Semen Citri Reticulatae (*Ju He*) and Folium Citri Reticulatae (*Ju Ye*). If there is breast distention and pain, add Fructus Meliae Toosendanis (*Chuan Lian Zi*) and Herba Cum Radice Taraxaci Mongolici (*Pu Gong Ying*). If there is breast distention with lumps, add Semen Vaccariae Segetalis (*Wang Bu Liu Xing*) and Squama Manitis (*Chuan Shan Jia*). If there is distention, lumps, and inflammation, add Herba Sargassi (*Hai Zao*) and Thallus Algae (*Kun Bu*). If there is kidney vacuity, add Cortex Eucommiae Ulmoidis (*Du Zhong*) and Radix Dipsaci (*Xu Duan*). If there is blood vacuity, add Radix Angelicae Sinensis (*Dang Gui*) and prepared Radix Rehmanniae (*Shu Di*). If there is vacuity cold of the *chong* and *ren*, add Gelatinum Cornu Cervi (*Lu Jiao Jiao*) and Cortex Cinnamomi (*Rou Gui*). For flaring fire, add Cortex Phellodendri (*Huang Bai*) and Herba Artemesiae Apiaciae (*Qing Hao*). And for dragging pain over the ovaries due to damp heat binding with qi and blood, add Radix Pulsatillae (*Bai Tou Weng*) and Caulis Sargentodoxae (*Hong Teng*).

---

[1] Zhu Xiao-nan, *Shanghai Lao Zhong Yi Jing Yan Xuan Bing (A Collection of Shanghai Old Masters' Clinical Experiences)*, ed. by Shanghai Municipal Health and Hygiene Office, Shanghai Science and Technology Press, Shanghai, 1984, p. 410-412

Xiang Fu Wan

Rhizoma Cyperi Rotundi (*Xiang Fu*)
Radix Angelicae Sinensis (*Dang Gui*)
Rhizoma Ligustici Wallichii (*Chuan Xiong*)
prepared Radix Rehmanniae (*Shu Di*)
wine-fried Radix Albus Paeoniae Lactiflorae (*Bai Shao*)
Rhizoma Alismatis (*Ze Xie*)
Pericarpium Citri Reticulatae (*Chen Pi*)
wine-fried Cortex Phellodendri (*Huang Bai*)
wine-fried Radix Glycyrrhizae (*Gan Cao*)

This formula courses the qi and strengthens the spleen, nourishes the blood and regulates the menses.

Zhong Zi Fang

Radix Angelicae Sinensis (*Dang Gui*)
Rhizoma Ligustici Wallichii (*Chuan Xiong*)
Fructus Evodiae Rutecarpae (*Wu Zhu*)
prepared Radix Rehmanniae (*Shu Di*)
processed Rhizoma Cyperi Rotundi (*Xiang Fu*)
Radix Albus Paeoniae Lactiflorae (*Bai Shao*)
Radix Salviae Miltiorrhizae (*Dan Shen*)
Sclerotium Poriae Cocoris (*Fu Ling*)
Pericarpium Citri Reticulatae (*Chen Pi*)
Rhizoma Corydalis Yanhusuo (*Yan Hu Suo*)

This formula courses the liver and rectifies the qi, quickens the blood and regulates the menses.

Tiao Jing Yu Zi Fang

wine-fried Radix Salviae Miltiorrhizae (*Dan Shen*)
Radix Angelicae Sinensis (*Dang Gui*)

Rhizoma Ligustici Wallichii (*Chuan Xiong*)
Radix Albus Paeoniae Lactiflorae (*Bai Shao*)
Radix Rehmanniae (*Gan Di*)
Pericarpium Citri Reticulatae (*Chen Pi*)
Pericarpium Viridis Citri Reticulatae (*Qing Pi*)
Rhizoma Cyperi Rotundi (*Xiang Fu*)
wine-fried Rhizoma Corydalis Yanhusuo (*Yan Hu*)
Flos Carthami Tinctorii (*Hong Hua*)

This formula's treatment principles are the same as the above.

Xiao Yu Li Qi Tang

Radix Angelicae Sinensis (*Dang Gui*)
Radix Salviae Miltiorrhizae (*Dan Shen*)
Radix Rubrus Paeoniae Lactiflorae (*Chi Shao*)
Rhizoma Cyperi Rotundi (*Xiang Fu*)
Radix Linderae Strychnifoliae (*Wu Yao*)
Radix Saussureae Seu Vladimiriae (*Guang Mu Xiang*)
Radix Dipsaci (*Xu Duan*)
Ramus Loranthi Seu Visci (*Sang Ji Sheng*)
stir-fried Cortex Eucommiae Ulmoidis (*Du Zhong*)
stir-fried Radix Cyathulae (*Chuan Niu Xi*)
Pericarpium Citri Reticulatae (*Chen Pi*)
Radix Glycyrrhizae (*Gan Cao*)

This formula is given by Guo Yuan for the treatment of infertility due to qi stagnation and blood stasis complicated by vacuity cold and low back and knee pain.

Xue Yu
Blood Stasis

Pathognomonic manifestations: Delayed menstruation, amount scant, color purplish black with blood clots and/or menstrual pain, possible

69

amenorrhea, lower abdominal pain which dislikes pressure, a dark, purple tongue or purple ecchymotic spots or patches on the tongue and especially the sides, and a fine, wiry, or choppy/astringent pulse

Therapeutic principles: Quicken the blood, transform stasis, and regulate the menses

Rx: *Xue Fu Zhu Yu Tang*

Semen Pruni Persicae (*Tao Ren*)
Flos Carthami Tinctorii (*Hong Hua*)
Radix Angelicae Sinensis (*Dang Gui*)
Rhizoma Ligustici Wallichii (*Chuan Xiong*)
Radix Rubrus Paeoniae Lactiflorae (*Chi Shao*)
Radix Cyathulae (*Chuan Niu Xi*)
Radix Bupleuri (*Chai Hu*)
Radix Platycodi Grandiflori (*Jie Geng*)
Fructus Citri Seu Ponciri (*Zhi Ke*)
Radix Rehmanniae (*Sheng Di*)
Radix Glycyrrhizae (*Gan Cao*)

The authors of *Zhong Yi Fu Chan Ke Xue (A Study of* TCM *Gynecology & Obstetrics)* recommend this formula for blood stasis infertility. Based on the ingredients in this formula, it is appropriate if there is an element of heat complicating this pattern.

Shao Fu Zhu Yu Tang

Radix Angelicae Sinensis (*Dang Gui*)
Rhizoma Ligustici Wallichii (*Chuan Xiong*)
Radix Rubrus Paeoniae Lactiflorae (*Chi Shao*)
Fructus Foeniculi Vulgaris (*Hui Xiang*)
Rhizoma Corydalis Yanhusuo (*Yan Hu Suo*)
Feces Trogopterori Seu Pteromi (*Wu Ling Zhi*)
Myrrha (*Mo Yao*)

Cortex Cinnamomi (*Rou Gui*)
Pollen Typhae (*Pu Huang*)
dry Rhizoma Zingiberis (*Gan Jiang*)

This standard prescription treats blood stasis complicated by an element of cold. For menstrual pain, Yeung Him-che says to delete dry Rhizoma Zingiberis and Cortex Cinnamomi and to add fresh Rhizoma Zingiberis (*Sheng Jiang*). This assumes that there is no cold complicating the case. For severe pain during menstruation, add Radix Saussureae Seu Vladimiriae (*Mu Xiang*) and Radix Albus Paeoniae Lactiflorae (*Bai Shao*). Wu and Qi suggest adding Herba Leonuri Heterophylli (*Yi Mu Cao*), Flos Carthami Tinctorii (*Hong Hua*), and Radix Cyathulae (*Chuan Niu Xi*). If there is abdominal distention and pain which dislike pressure, add Rhizoma Sparganii (*San Leng*), Rhizoma Curcumae Zedoariae (*E Zhu*), and Semen Vaccariae Segetalis (*Wang Bu Liu Xing*). If menstrual pain is severe, add Radix Bupleuri (*Chai Hu*), Rhizoma Cyperi Rotundi (*Xiang Fu*), and Fructus Meliae Toosendanis (*Chuan Lian Zi*). If there is stasis with simultaneous vacuity, add Radix Astragali Membranacei (*Huang Qi*), stir-fried Cortex Eucommiae Ulmoidis (*Du Zhong*), and Plastrum Testudinis (*Gui Ban*).

Jia Jian Shao Fu Zhu Yu Tang

Radix Rubrus Paeoniae Lactiflorae (*Chi Shao*)
Radix Angelicae Sinensis (*Dang Gui*)
Pollen Typhae (*Pu Huang*)
Fructus Liquidambaris Taiwaniae (*Lu Lu Tong*)
Feces Trogopterori Seu Pteromi (*Wu Ling Zhi*)
Radix Salviae Miltiorrhizae (*Dan Shen*)
Rhizoma Ligustici Wallichii (*Chuan Xiong*)
blast-fried Squama Manitis (*Shan Jia*)
Flos Carthami Tinctorii (*Hong Hua*)
Rhizoma Corydalis Yanhusuo (*Yan Hu Suo*)
Myrrha (*Mo Yao*)

71

If there is prominent heat as evidenced by excessive, malodorous abnormal vaginal discharge accompanied by palpable swelling and lump with pain upon pressure, add Herba Patriniae Heterophyllae (*Bai Jiang Cao*), Cortex Radicis Moutan (*Dan Pi*), Semen Pruni Persicae (*Tao Ren*), and Herba Cum Radice Taraxaci Mongolici (*Pu Gong Ying*). If there is chilly pain in the lower abdomen, add Fructus Evodiae Rutecarpae (*Wu Zhu Yu*), Cortex Cinnamomi (*Rou Gui*), and blast-fried Rhizoma Zingiberis (*Pao Jiang*). If there is low back pain, add Radix Dipsaci (*Xu Duan*), Ramus Loranthi Seu Visci (*Sang Ji Sheng*), and Radix Achyranthis Bidentatae (*Niu Xi*). During the period, delete Myrrha and Cortex Radicis Moutan.

Kai Yu Zhong Yu Tang Jia Jian

Radix Angelicae Sinensis (*Dang Gui*)
Radix Rubrus Paeoniae Lactiflorae (*Chi Shao*)
Rhizoma Cyperi Rotundi (*Xiang Fu*)
Fructus Liquidambaris Taiwaniae (*Lu Lu Tong*)
Radix Rubiae Cordifoliae (*Qian Cao*)
Semen Pruni Persicae (*Tao Ren*)
Flos Carthami Tinctorii (*Hong Hua*)
Pollen Typhae (*Pu Huang*)
Caulis Sargentodoxae (*Hong Teng*)
Fructus Citri Seu Ponciri (*Zhi Ke*)
Spina Gleditschiae Chinensis (*Jiao Ci*)
Herba Salviae Chinensis (*Shi Jian Chuan*)
Herba Epimedii (*Xian Ling Pi*)

Shen Chong-li recommends this formula for qi stagnation, blood stasis infertility. It is to be administered after the menses ceases and during the premenstruum.

Tao Hong Si Wu Tang Jia Jian

Semen Pruni Persicae (*Tao Ren*)

Flos Carthami Tinctorii (*Hong Hua*)
Radix Angelicae Sinensis (*Dang Gui*)
Rhizoma Ligustici Wallichii (*Chuan Xiong*)
Radix Rubrus Paeoniae Lactiflorae (*Chi Shao*)
Rhizoma Curcumae Zedoariae (*E Zhu*)
Rhizoma Corydalis Yanhusuo (*Yan Hu Suo*)
Radix Linderae Strychnifoliae (*Wu Yao*)
Rhizoma Cyperi Rotundi (*Xiang Fu*)
Radix Salviae Miltiorrhizae (*Dan Shen*)

If abdominal pain is ameliorated by warmth, add Fructus Foeniculi
Vulgaris (*Xiao Hui Xiang*) and Folium Artemesiae Argyii (*Ai Ye*). If
the fallopian tubes are blocked, add Spina Gleditschiae Chinensis
(*Jiao Ci*), and stir-fried Squama Manitis (*Chuan Jia*). In case of
pelvic inflammation with palpable lumps in the lower abdomen and
recurrent pain, add Caulis Milletiae Seu Spatholobi (*Ji Xue Teng*),
Fructus Forsythiae Suspensae (*Lian Qiao*), and Rhizoma Sparganii
(*San Leng*).

Unnamed formula given in *Concise Traditional Chinese Gynecology*

Radix Angelicae Sinensis (*Dang Gui*)
Radix Rubrus Paeoniae Lactiflorae (*Chi Shao*)
Rhizoma Corydalis Yanhusuo (*Yan Hu Suo*)
Lignum Sappanis (*Su Mu*)
Retinervus Fructi Luffae (*Si Gua Lou*)

Unnamed formula given by Shang Xian-ming *et al.*

Radix Angelicae Sinensis (*Dang Gui*)
Rhizoma Ligustici Wallichii (*Chuan Xiong*)
Radix Salviae Miltiorrhizae (*Dan Shen*)
Semen Pruni Persicae (*Tao Ren*)
Squama Manitis (*Shan Jia*)

Ramulus Ilicis Chinensis (*Dong Qing*)
Fructus Liquidambaris Taiwanensis (*Lu Lu Tong*)
Spina Gleditschiae (*Jiao Ci*)
Herba Sargassi (*Hai Zao*)
Sanguis Draconis (*Xue Jie*)
Radix Bupleuri (*Chai Hu*)
Radix Saussureae Seu Vladimiriae (*Mu Xiang*)

Shang Xian-ming *et al.* say that this formula treats stagnant qi and blood stasis resulting in obstruction of the fallopian tubes.

Unnamed formula given by Wu and Qi

Radix Angelicae Sinensis (*Dang Gui*)
Rhizoma Ligustici Wallichii (*Chuan Xiong*)
Radix Albus Paeoniae Lactiflorae (*Bai Shao*)
dry Rhizoma Zingiberis (*Gan Jiang*)
Tuber Curcumae (*Yu Jin*)
Semen Cuscutae (*Tu Si Zi*)
Flos Carthami Tinctorii (*Hong Hua*)
Cortex Cinnamomi (*Rou Gui*)

Wu and Qi say to administer this formula during the menstruation.

Tiao Jing Zhong Zi Shen Xiao Fang

Radix Salviae Miltiorrhizae (*Dan Shen*)
Rhizoma Cyperi Rotundi (*Xiang Fu*)
Radix Angelicae Sinensis (*Dang Gui*)
Rhizoma Ligustici Wallichii (*Chuan Xiong*)
Radix Albus Paeoniae Lactiflorae (*Bai Shao*)
Cortex Radicis Moutan (*Dan Pi*)
Herba Leonuri Heterophylli (*Yi Mu Cao*)

This formula treats qi stagnation and blood stasis. Some Chinese *fu ke* texts discuss this as a single category, *qi zhi xue yu*.

Zhong Yu Wan

Herba Leonuri Heterophylli (*Yi Mu Cao*)
Rhizoma Ligustici Wallichii (*Chuan Xiong*)
Radix Rubrus Paeoniae Lactiflorae (*Chi Shao*)
Radix Angelicae Sinensis (*Dang Gui*)
Radix Saussureae Seu Vladimiriae (*Guang Mu Xiang*)

Gui Zhi Fu Ling Wan

Ramulus Cinnamomi (*Gui Zhi*)
Sclerotium Poriae Cocoris (*Fu Ling*)
Radix Rubrus Paeoniae Lactiflorae (*Chi Shao*)
Cortex Radicis Moutan (*Dan Pi*)
Semen Pruni Persicae (*Tao Ren*)

Yeung Him-che simply gives this formula for the treatment of blood stasis infertility. Hong-yen Hsu also recommends this formula for blood stasis infertility in a woman with a moderately strong build and darkish complexion for whom *Tao He Cheng Qi Tang* is too strong.

Gui Zhi Fu Ling Wan Jia Wei

Ramulus Cinnamomi (*Gui Zhi*)
Sclerotium Poriae Cocoris (*Fu Ling*)
Radix Rubrus Paeoniae Lactiflorae (*Chi Shao*)
Cortex Radicis Moutan (*Dan Pi*)
Semen Pruni Persicae (*Tao Ren*)
Flos Carthami Tinctorii (*Hong Hua*)
Radix Salviae Miltiorrhizae (*Dan Shen*)
Rhizoma Sparganii (*San Leng*)
Rhizoma Curcumae Zedoariae (*E Zhu*)

This is Huang Shou-ren's modification. He says to use this formula for infertility due to blood stasis manifest by abdominal pain when the period comes. This is based on the principles of warming the channels/menses and transforming stasis.

Tao He Cheng Qi Tang

Semen Pruni Persicae (*Tao Ren*)
Ramulus Cinnamomi (*Gui Zhi*)
Radix Et Rhizoma Rhei (*Da Huang*)
Mirabilitum (*Mang Xiao*)
mix-fried Radix Glycyrrhizae (*Zhi Gan Cao*)

This formula is given by Hong-yen Hsu for the treatment of blood stasis infertility in an obese, replete patient with constipation. If blood stasis is severe, add Radix Angelicae Sinensis (*Dang Gui*) and Flos Carthami Tinctorii (*Hong Hua*). If qi stagnation accompanies this condition, add Rhizoma Cyperi Rotundi (*Xiang Fu*) and Pericarpium Viridis Citri Reticulatae (*Qing Pi*). Yeung Him-che says this formula is appropriate when there is heat and blood stasis. Hong-yen Hsu corroborates this but says that there is heat above but cold below. This explains the Ramulus Cinnamomi beyond its just promoting the flow of qi and blood in the channels and connecting vessels since it also returns yang to its lower source. (This may also apply to *Gui Zhi Fu Ling Wan* as well.) The other signs and symptoms Hsu gives for this formula are flushing up, dizziness, and constipation, while Yeung gives acute abdominal pain, thirst, a dry mouth, increased body temperature at night, a red, dry tongue, and a deep, forceful or grating/astringent pulse.

Another way of seeing all of the last three formulas is that they address yin fire with blood stasis. There is dampness and cold below but heat in the blood level which tends to flush upwards. Except for this complication of heat in the *xue fen*, any of these formulas might also be placed in the following category.

Han Shi Cheng Jing
Cold Dampness Accumulating in the Channels

Pathognomonic manifestations: Delayed menses or prolonged menstrual flow, amount scant, color dark purplish with clots, chilly pain in the lower abdomen relieved somewhat by warmth, a thin, white abnormal vaginal discharge, a dull colored tongue with thin, white coating, and a deep, slow pulse

Song and Yu call this pattern cold uterus or *gong han*. Some books lump it under kidney yang vacuity. In this case, there is blood stasis aggravated by obstruction from cold and damp evils.

Therapeutic principles: Warm the uterus and scatter cold

Rx: *Ai Fu Nuan Gong Wan*

Folium Artemesiae Argyii (*Ai Ye*)
Rhizoma Cyperi Rotundi (*Xiang Fu*)
Radix Angelicae Sinensis (*Dang Gui*)
Radix Dipsaci (*Xu Duan*)
Fructus Corni Officinalis (*Shan Zhu Yu*)
Rhizoma Ligustici Wallichii (*Chuan Xiong*)
Radix Albus Paeoniae Lactiflorae (*Bai Shao*)
Radix Astragali Membranacei (*Huang Qi*)
prepared Radix Rehmanniae (*Shu Di*)
Cortex Cinnamomi (*Rou Gui*)

This formula given by Song and Yu is extremely similar in composition to many of those appearing under the kidney yang vacuity category above.

Shao Fu Zhu Yu Tang Jia Jian #1

stir-fried Fructus Foeniculi Vulgaris (*Xiao Hui Xiang*)

Cortex Cinnamomi (*Gui Pi*)
Fructus Evodiae Rutecarpae (*Wu Zhu Yu*)
Radix Linderae Strychnifoliae (*Wu Yao*)
Herba Epimedii (*Xian Ling Pi*)
Radix Angelicae Sinensis (*Dang Gui*)
Rhizoma Ligustici Wallichii (*Chuan Xiong*)
Pollen Typhae (*Pu Huang*)
Feces Trogopterori Seu Pteromi (*Wu Ling Zhi*)
Radix Rubrus Paeoniae Lactiflorae (*Chi Shao*)
Rhizoma Corydalis Yanhusuo (*Yan Hu Suo*)
Rhizoma Atractylodis (*Cang Zhu*)
blast-fried Rhizoma Zingiberis (*Pao Jiang*)

A different version of this formula appears above under the blood stasis category.

Shao Fu Zhu Yu Tang Jia Jian #2

Radix Angelicae Sinensis (*Dang Gui*)
Fructus Foeniculi Vulgaris (*Xiao Hui Xiang*)
Rhizoma Corydalis Yanhusuo (*Yuan Hu*)
Rhizoma Ligustici Wallichii (*Chuan Xiong*)
blast-fried Rhizoma Zingiberis (*Pao Jiang*)
Pollen Typhae (*Sheng Pu Huang*)
Cortex Cinnamomi (*Guan Gui*)
Radix Rubrus Paeoniae Lactiflorae (*Chi Shao*)
Feces Trogopterori Seu Pteromi (*Wu Ling Zhi*)
Herba Epimedii (*Xian Ling Pi*)
Herba Leonuri Heterophylli (*Yi Mu Cao*)

This is yet again another version of this formula given by Sun Jiu-ling for cold dampness congealing and stagnating.

Wen Jing Tang

Fructus Evodiae Rutecarpae (*Wu Zhu Yu*)
Ramulus Cinnamomi (*Gui Zhi*)
Radix Angelicae Sinensis (*Dang Gui*)
Rhizoma Ligustici Wallichii (*Chuan Xiong*)
Radix Albus Paeoniae Lactiflorae (*Bai Shao*)
Gelatinum Corii Asini (*E Jiao*)
Tuber Ophiopogonis Japonicae (*Mai Dong*)
Cortex Radicis Moutan (*Dan Pi*)
Radix Panacis Ginseng (*Ren Shen*)
Rhizoma Pinelliae Ternatae (*Ban Xia*)
fresh Rhizoma Zingiberis (*Sheng Jiang*)
Radix Glycyrrhizae (*Gan Cao*)

Yeung Him-che suggests this formula for infertility due to accumulation of cold in the channels. It should be remembered that the character for channels, *jing*, also means the menses. If chilly pain of the lower abdomen is severe, delete Tuber Ophiopogonis Japonicae and Cortex Radicis Moutan, add Fructus Foeniculi Vulgaris (*Xiao Hui Xiang*) and Folium Artemesiae Argyii (*Ai Ye*), and substitute Cortex Cinnamomi (*Rou Gui*) for Ramulus Cinnamomi. If qi stagnation is prominent, add Rhizoma Cyperi Rotundi (*Xiang Fu*) and Radix Linderae Strychnifoliae (*Wu Yao*). For more pronounced qi vacuity, add Radix Astragali Membranacei (*Huang Qi*). And for infertility due to blood vacuity and cold, add Pericarpium Viridis Citri Reticulatae (*Qing Pi*) and Rhizoma Cyperi Rotundi (*Xiang Fu*).

According to Bensky and Barolet, this formula was originally devised for treating vacuity cold entering the *chong* and *ren* with internal obstruction due to blood stasis. Going back to the *Jin Gui Yao Lue (Essential Prescriptions From the Golden Cabinet)*, one sees it was prescribed for a menopausal woman with *lou xia* and fever at dusk. This is clearly a case of hot above and cold below. In the lower burner there is vacuity cold and blood stasis. Rootless yang, however flushes upward steaming the heart and lungs. This then accounts for the Cortex Radicis Moutan and Tuber Ophiopogonis. Ramulus

Cinnamomi and Fructus Evodiae Rutecarpae not only warm the channels and quicken the blood but also redirect yang qi downwards. This downward redirection is aided by Rhizoma Pinelliae Ternatae. This scenario of hot above but cold below is a commonly encountered one in Western infertility patients who are in their late thirties and early forties. As I have discussed in *My Sister the Moon*, it is also a commonly encountered pattern in women who have suffered sexual abuse.

Wen Jing San Han

Fructus Foeniculi Vulgaris (*Xiao Hui*)
dry Rhizoma Zingiberis (*Gan Jiang*)
Rhizoma Corydalis Yanhusuo (*Yan Hu Suo*)
Radix Angelicae Sinensis (*Dang Gui*)
Myrrha (*Mo Yao*)
Rhizoma Ligustici Wallichii (*Chuan Xiong*)
Cortex Cinnamomi (*Guan Gui*)
Radix Rubrus Paeoniae Lactiflorae (*Chi Shao*)
Feces Trogopterori Seu Pteromi (*Wu Ling Zhi*)
Pollen Typhae (*Pu Huang*)

Tan Shi Zu Zhi
Phlegm Dampness Blockage & Stagnation

Pathognomonic manifestations: Infertility, a fat or obese body, excessive phlegm production, delayed menstruation or amenorrhea, chest oppression, abdominal distention, excessive, white vaginal discharge, dizziness, lack of strength, heaviness of the four limbs, possible swelling and edema of the lower limbs, facial color white, heart palpitations, a tendency to nausea, a white, slimy tongue coating, and a slippery; soggy and thready; or thready and relaxed/retarded pulse

Therapeutic principles: Eliminate dampness, transform phlegm, and regulate the menses

Rx: *Qi Gong Wan*

processed Rhizoma Pinelliae Ternatae (*Ban Xia*)
Rhizoma Atractylodis (*Cang Zhu*)
Rhizoma Cyperi Rotundi (*Xiang Fu*)
Massa Medica Fermentata (*Shen Qu*)
Sclerotium Poriae Cocoris (*Fu Ling*)
Pericarpium Citri Reticulatae (*Chen Pi*)
Rhizoma Ligustici Wallichii (*Chuan Xiong*)

Luo Yuan-qi *et al.*, compilers of *Zhong Yi Fu Ke Xue (A Study of TCM Gynecology)*, say to regularly add Rhizoma Acori Graminei (*Shi Chang Pu*). Then, if there are heart palpitations, add Radix Polygalae Tenuifoliae (*Yuan Zhi*). If the menses is excessive in amount, delete Rhizoma Ligustici Wallichii and add Radix Astragali Membranacei (*Huang Qi*) and Radix Dipsaci (*Xu Duan*) to boost the qi and consolidate the kidneys. Likewise, Zhang En-qin *et al.* also say to add Rhizoma Acori Graminei to the above formula but then also add Herba Sargassi (*Hai Zao*) and Thallus Algae (*Kun Bu*).

Jia Wei Qi Gong Wan

Rhizoma Pinelliae Ternatae (*Ban Xia*)
Rhizoma Atractylodis (*Cang Zhu*)
Rhizoma Cyperi Rotundi (*Xiang Fu*)
Cornu Cervi (*Lu Jiao*)
Rhizoma Ligustici Wallichii (*Chuan Xiong*)
Pericarpium Citri Reticulatae (*Chen Pi*)
Sclerotium Poriae Cocoris (*Fu Ling*)
Massa Medica Fermentata (*Shen Qu*)
Herba Epimedii (*Yin Yang Huo*)

81

Bu Shen Hua Shi Tang

prepared Radix Rehmanniae (*Shu Di*)
Semen Cuscutae (*Tu Si Zi*)
Fructus Rubi (*Fu Pen Zi*)
Rhizoma Curculiginis Orchoidis (*Xian Mao*)
Herba Epimedii (*Xian Ling Pi*)
Spica Prunellae Vulgaris (*Xia Gu Cao*)
Squama Manitis (*Shan Jia*)
Thallus Algae (*Kun Bu*)
Bulbus Fritillariae Thunbergii (*Bei Mu*)
Semen Plantaginis (*Che Qian Zi*)

This formula warms the kidneys and strengthens yang, transforms phlegm and dispels dampness.

Xiao Zhi Mo Dao Tan Tang

processed Rhizoma Pinelliae Ternatae (*Ban Xia*)
blast-fried Rhizoma Arisaematis (*Nan Xing*)
Pericarpium Citri Erythrocarpae (*Ju Hong*)
Fructus Citri Seu Ponciri (*Zhi Ke*)
Sclerotium Poriae Cocoris (*Fu Ling*)
Talcum (*Hua Shi*)
Rhizoma Ligustici Wallichii (*Chuan Xiong*)
Radix Ledebouriellae Sesloidis (*Fang Feng*)
Radix Et Rhizoma Notopterygii (*Qiang Huo*)
Semen Plantaginis (*Che Qian Zi*)

This formula strengthens the spleen and transforms dampness, rectifies the qi and transforms phlegm.

Cang Fu Dao Tan Wan

Rhizoma Atractylodis (*Cang Zhu*)

Rhizoma Cyperi Rotundi (*Xiang Fu*)
Pericarpium Citri Reticulatae (*Chen Pi*)
Sclerotium Poriae Cocoris (*Fu Ling*)
Fructus Citri Seu Ponciri (*Zhi Qiao*)
processed Rhizoma Pinelliae Ternatae (*Ban Xia*)
processed Rhizoma Arisaematis (*Nan Xing*)
mix-fried Radix Glycyrrhizae (*Zhi Gan Cao*)
fresh Rhizoma Zingiberis (*Sheng Jiang*)

This formula is from *Ye Tian Shi Nu Ke (Ye Tian-shi's Gynecology)*. Wu and Qi suggest adding Rhizoma Ligustici Wallichii (*Chuan Xiong*), Radix Achyranthis Bidentatae (*Niu Xi*), and Herba Leonuri Heterophylli (*Yi Mu Cao*).

Cang Fu Dao Tan Wan Jia Jian #1

processed Rhizoma Cyperi Rotundi (*Xiang Fu*)
stir-fried Rhizoma Ligustici Wallichii (*Chuan Xiong*)
Pericarpium Citri Erythrocarpae (*Guang Ju Hong*)
Sclerotium Poriae Cocoris (*Fu Ling*)
ginger-processed Rhizoma Pinelliae Ternatae (*Jiang Ban Xia*)
scorched Massa Medica Fermentata (*Shen Qu*)
mix-fried Radix Glycyrrhizae (*Zhi Gan Cao*)
Rhizoma Acori Graminei (*Gan Chang Pu*)
Rhizoma Atractylodis (*Cang Zhu*)
Radix Angelicae Sinensis (*Quan Dang Gui*)

Shi Cheng-han says to take 7-10 *ji* of this formula before menstruation followed by the following two pills after menstruation.

Cang Fu Dao Tan Wan Jia Jian #2

Rhizoma Atractylodis (*Cang Zhu*)
Rhizoma Cyperi Rotundi (*Xiang Fu*)
Fructus Citri Seu Ponciri (*Zhi Ke*)

Sclerotium Poriae Cocoris (*Fu Ling*)
Rhizoma Arisaematis (*Nan Xing*)
Pericarpium Citri Reticulatae (*Chen Pi*)
processed Rhizoma Pinelliae Ternatae (*Ban Xia*)
Rhizoma Ligustici Wallichii (*Chuan Xiong*)
Rhizoma Acori Graminei (*Chang Pu*)
Herba Epimedii (*Xian Ling Pi*)
Semen Cuscutae (*Tu Si Zi*)
Semen Vaccariae Segetalis (*Wang Bu Liu Xing*)
Fluoritum (*Zi Shi Ying*)
fresh Fructus Crataegi (*Shan Zha*)

This version is given by Shen Chong-li. It not only transforms phlegm and eliminates dampness but also warms yang and supplements the kidneys based on modern Chinese ideas concerning female infertility. Shen says to administer this formula after the menses.

Jia Wei Cang Fu Dao Tan Wan

Sclerotium Poriae Cocoris (*Fu ling*)
Rhizoma Pinelliae Ternatae (*Ban Xia*)
Pericarpium Citri Reticulatae (*Chen Pi*)
Radix Glycyrrhizae (*Gan Cao*)
Rhizoma Cyperi Rotundi (*Xiang Fu*)
Rhizoma Atractylodis (*Cang Zhu*)
processed Rhizoma Arisaematis (*Nan Xing*)
Fructus Immaturus Citri Seu Ponciri (*Zhi Shi*)
Radix Codonopsis Pilosulae (*Dang Shen*)
fresh Rhizoma Zingiberis (*Sheng Jiang*)
Radix Morindae Officinalis (*Ba Ji Tian*)
Herba Epimedii (*Yin Yang Huo*)
Pulvis Cornu Cervi (*Lu Rong Fen*)

This version of this formula, given by Wang and Wang in *Fu Ke Lin Chuang Jing Hua (The Essence of Clinical Gynecology)*, with its inclusion of kidney-supplementing ingredients is likewise predicated upon the modern TCM notion that kidney vacuity is a part of most female infertility.

Cang Zhu Dao Tan Wan Jia Wei

Rhizoma Atractylodis (*Cang Zhu*)
Pericarpium Citri Reticulatae (*Chen Pi*)
Sclerotium Poriae Cocoris (*Fu Ling*)
Fructus Citri Seu Ponciri (*Zhi Ke*)
Rhizoma Pinelliae Ternatae (*Fa Xia*)
Caulis Bambusae In Taeniis (*Zhu Ru*)
Thallus Algae (*Kun Bu*)
Herba Sargassi (*Hai Zao*)
Rhizoma Acori Graminei (*Shi Chang Pu*)

Liu and Liu suggest deleting Rhizoma Ligustici Wallichii and adding Radix Astragali Membranacei (*Huang Qi*) and Radix Dipsaci (*Xu Duan*) in order to boost the qi and consolidate the kidneys if the menstrual flow is excessive. If there are heart palpitations, they recommend adding Radix Polygalae Tenuifoliae (*Yuan Zhi*) to tranquilize the heart.

Zao Shi Huo Tan Fang

stir-fried Rhizoma Atractylodis (*Cang Zhu*)
stir-fried Rhizoma Atractylodis Macrocephalae (*Bai Zhu*)
Concretio Silicea Bambusae (*Tian Zhu Huang*)
ginger-processed Rhizoma Pinelliae Ternatae (*Ban Xia*)
Retinervus Fructi Citri (*Ju Luo*)
Pollen Typhae (*Pu Huang*)
Rhizoma Curcumae Zedoariae (*E Zhu*)
Rhizoma Acori Graminei (*Shi Chang Pu*)
gall-processed Rhizoma Arisaematis (*Nan Xing*)
Fructus Citri Seu Ponciri (*Zhi Ke*)

Caulis Bambusae In Taeniis (*Zhu Ru*)
Sclerotium Poriae Cocoris (*Fu Ling*)

In case of shortness of breath and excessive abnormal vaginal discharge, add Radix Codonopsis Pilosulae (*Dang Shen*), Radix Astragali Membranacei (*Huang Qi*), and Radix Albus Paeoniae Lactiflorae (*Bai Shao*). If the menses is delayed and scant, add Herba Epimedii (*Xian Ling Pi*), Radix Dipsaci (*Xu Duan*), and Radix Angelicae Sinensis (*Dang Gui*).

Er Chen Wan

Rhizoma Pinelliae Ternatae (*Ban Xia*)
Pericarpium Citri Reticulatae (*Chen Pi*)
Sclerotium Poriae Cocoris (*Fu Ling*)
Radix Glycyrrhizae (*Gan Cao*)

The authors of *Zhong Yi Fu Chan Ke Xue (The Study of* TCM *Gynecology & Obstetrics)* recommend adding Rhizoma Arisaematis (*Nan Xing*) and Rhizoma Atractylodis (*Cang Zhu*) to transform phlegm, fortify the spleen, and dry dampness, Rhizoma Cyperi Rotundi (*Xiang Fu*) and Fructus Immaturus Citri Seu Ponciri (*Zhi Shi*) to move the qi, and fresh Rhizoma Zingiberis (*Sheng Jiang*) to scatter cold.

Yue Ju Wan

Rhizoma Atractylodis (*Cang Zhu*)
Rhizoma Ligustici Wallichii (*Chuan Xiong*)
Rhizoma Cyperi Rotundi (*Xiang Fu*)
Fructus Gardeniae Jasminoidis (*Zhi Zi*)
Massa Medica Fermentata (*Shen Qu*)

Bu Zhong Yi Qi Tang Jia Wei

Radix Astragali Membranacei (*Huang Qi*)
Radix Codonopsis Pilosulae (*Dang Shen*)
Radix Angelicae Sinensis (*Dang Gui*)
stir-fried Rhizoma Atractylodis Macrocephalae (*Bai Zhu*)
Radix Glycyrrhizae (*Gan Cao*)
Rhizoma Cimicifugae (*Sheng Ma*)
Radix Bupleuri (*Chai Hu*)
Sclerotium Poriae Cocoris (*Fu Ling*)
Pericarpium Citri Reticulatae (*Chen Pi*)
Rhizoma Pinelliae Ternatae (*Ban Xia*)

Unnamed formula from *Concise Traditional Chinese Gynecology*

processed Rhizoma Pinelliae Ternatae (*Ban Xia*)
fried Rhizoma Atractylodis (*Cang Zhu*)
Sclerotium Poriae Cocoris (*Fu Ling*)
processed Rhizoma Cyperi Rotundi (*Xiang Fu*)
Rhizoma Ligustici Wallichii (*Chuan Xiong*)

Unnamed formula given by Shang Xian-ming *et al.*

Fructus Crataegi (*Shan Zha*)
Rhizoma Curculiginis Orchoidis (*Xian Mao*)
Herba Epimedii (*Xian Ling Pi*)
Semen Cuscutae (*Tu Si Zi*)
Fructus Rubi (*Fu Pen Zi*)
Rhizoma Arisaematis (*Nan Xing*)
Rhizoma Pinelliae Ternatae (*Ban Xia*)
Sclerotium Poriae Cocoris (*Fu Ling*)
processed Rhizoma Cyperi Rotundi (*Xiang Fu*)
Fructus Citri Seu Ponciri (*Zhi Ke*)
Rhizoma Atractylodis Macrocephalae (*Bai Zhu*)
Rhizoma Ligustici Wallichii (*Chuan Xiong*)
Herba Lycopi Lucidi (*Ze Lan*)

Shang Xian-ming *et al.* give the following two unnamed formulas for the treatment of phlegm damp retention obstructing the channels with kidney qi insufficiency, obesity, and hirsutism:

Herba Epimedii (*Xian Ling Pi*)
Radix Morindae Officinalis (*Ba Ji Tian*)
Cornu Parvum Cervi (*Lu Rong*)
Semen Cuscutae (*Tu Si Zi*)
Radix Dioscoreae Oppositae (*Shan Yao*)
Rhizoma Atractylodis (*Cang Zhu*)
Rhizoma Atractylodis Macrocephalae (*Bai Zhu*)
Semen Sinapis Albae (*Bai Jie Zi*)
processed Rhizoma Cyperi Rotundi (*Xiang Fu*)
Radix Angelicae Sinensis (*Dang Gui*)
Rhizoma Acori Graminei (*Shi Chang Pu*)
Rhizoma Arisaematis (*Nan Xing*)
Herba Sargassi (*Hai Zao*)
Herba Leonuri Heterophylli (*Yi Mu Cao*)

Administer 1 *ji* per day from days 5-11 of the menstrual cycle.

Radix Angelicae Sinensis (*Dang Gui*)
Radix Salviae Miltiorrhizae (*Dan Shen*)
Rhizoma Ligustici Wallichii (*Chuan Xiong*)
Radix Rubrus Paeoniae Lactiflorae (*Chi Shao*)
Herba Artemesiae Anomalae (*Liu Ji Nu*)
Caulis Milletiae Seu Spatholobi (*Ji Xue Teng*)
Herba Lycopi Lucidi (*Ze Lan*)
processed Rhizoma Cyperi Rotundi (*Xiang Fu*)
Herba Leonuri Heterophylli (*Yi Mu Cao*)
Flos Carthami Tinctorii (*Hong Hua*)
Cortex Cinnamomi (*Gui Pi*)
Spina Gleditschiae Chinensis (*Jiao Ci*)

Administer 1 *ji* per day from days 12-18 of the menstrual cycle.

Unnamed formula given by Wu and Qi

Pericarpium Citri Reticulatae (*Chen Pi*)
ginger-fried Rhizoma Pinelliae Ternatae (*Ban Xia*)
Sclerotium Poriae Cocoris (*Fu Ling*)
Sclerotium Polypori Umbellati (*Zhu Ling*)
Ramulus Cinnamomi (*Gui Zhi*)
Fructus Immaturus Citri Seu Ponciri (*Zhi Shi*)
Rhizoma Arisaematis (*Nan Xing*)
Rhizoma Alismatis (*Ze Xie*)
Herba Leonuri Heterophylli (*Yi Mu Cao*)
Radix Glycyrrhizae (*Sheng Gan Cao*)

Unnamed formula given by He and Jiang

Radix Angelicae Sinensis (*Dang Gui*)
Sclerotium Poriae Cocoris (*Fu Ling*)
Rhizoma Ligustici Wallichii (*Chuan Xiong*)
Radix Albus Paeoniae Lactiflorae (*Bai Shao*)
Rhizoma Atractylodis Macrocephalae (*Bai Zhu*)
Rhizoma Pinelliae Ternatae (*Ban Xia*)
Rhizoma Cyperi Rotundi (*Xiang Fu*)
Pericarpium Citri Reticulatae (*Chen Pi*)
Radix Glycyrrhizae (*Gan Cao*)
Massa Medica Fermentata (*Shen Qu*)

He and Jiang say to use this formula for infertility due to obesity.

Another unnamed formula from He and Jiang

Rhizoma Pinelliae Ternatae (*Ban Xia*)
Rhizoma Atractylodis (*Cang Zhu*)
Rhizoma Cyperi Rotundi (*Xiang Fu*)
Massa Medica Fermentata (*Shen Qu*)
Sclerotium Poriae Cocoris (*Fu Ling*)

Pericarpium Citri Reticulatae (*Chen Pi*)
Rhizoma Ligustici Wallichii (*Chuan Xiong*)
Herba Sargassi (*Hai Zao*)
Thallus Algae (*Kun Bu*)
Rhizoma Acori Graminei (*Shi Chang Pu*)

Zhong Zi Miao Fang

Fructus Evodiae Rutecarpae (*Wu Zhu Yu*)
stir-fried Radix Aconiti Carmichaeli (*Bai Fu Zi*)
Cortex Cinnamomi (*Gui Xin*)
Radix Panacis Ginseng (*Ren Shen*)
Pericarpium Citri Reticulatae (*Chen Pi*)
Sclerotium Poriae Cocoris (*Fu Ling*)
Fructus Schizandrae Chinensis (*Wu Wei Zi*)
Rhizoma Acori Graminei (*Shi Chang Pu*)
Radix Angelicae (*Bai Zhi*)
Radix Ampelopsis (*Bai Lian*)
Cortex Magnoliae Officinalis (*Hou Po*)
Radix Angelicae Sinensis (*Dang Gui*)
Radix Achyranthis Bidentatae (*Niu Xi*)
Herba Cum Radice Asari Seiboldi (*Xi Xin*)
Gummum Olibani (*Ru Xiang*)
Myrrha (*Mo Yao*)

According to Du Jie-hui, this formula warms the channels and transforms phlegm, regulates the menses and promotes fertility. It might just as easily have been put under the cold uterus category complicated by phlegm and dampness.

Xue Yu Shi Re
Blood Stasis & Damp Heat

Pathognomonic manifestations: Early menses, amount scant, color purplish red with clots, lower abdominal distention and pain, especially along the sides of the abdomen, which dislikes pressure, or stabbing pain in the lower abdomen, breast distention and pain, chest and flank distention and pain, abdominal pain aggravated as the period draws near, body emaciated, chronic lumbar soreness, possible low fever, possible abnormal vaginal discharge which is yellow and foul smelling, a red tongue with a thin, yellow coating, and a wiry, rapid pulse

Song and Yu call this pattern stasis heat (*yu re*). It is a combination of dampness and heat in the lower burner wrestling and knotting with stagnant qi and blood stasis. Depending upon the prevalence of these four elements in this scenario, the signs and symptoms may vary somewhat from patient to patient. This pattern is often overlooked in Chinese *fu ke* texts and is often misdiagnosed in clinical practice since it includes elements of blood stasis, qi stagnation, damp heat, and seeming yin vacuity. It may also even include an element of kidney yang vacuity and cold as well since, according to Li Dong-yuan, damp heat in the intestines impairs the source of transformation of kidney yang.

Therapeutic principles: Clear heat and eliminate dampness, quicken the blood and dispel stasis

Rx: *Qing Re Xiao Yu Tang*

Radix Angelicae Sinensis (*Dang Gui*)
scorched Radix Albus Paeoniae Lactiflorae (*Bai Shao*)
Fructus Meliae Toosendanis (*Chuan Lian Zi*)
Radix Bupleuri (*Chai Hu*)
Caulis Sargentodoxae (*Hong Teng*)
Rhizoma Corydalis Yanhusuo (*Yan Hu Suo*)
stir-fried Fructus Citri Seu Ponciri (*Zhi Qiao*)
Tuber Curcumae (*Guang Yu Jin*)
Herba Menthae (*Bo He*)
Talcum (*Hua Shi*)

Radix Glycyrrhizae (*Gan Cao*)

Tiao Gan Pi Tang He Chuan Lian Zi San Jia Jian

Radix Bupleuri (*Chai Hu*)
Fructus Immaturus Citri Seu Ponciri (*Zhi Shi*)
Radix Rubrus Paeoniae Lactiflorae (*Chi Shao*)
Radix Glycyrrhizae (*Gan Cao*)
Rhizoma Corydalis Yanhusuo (*Yan Hu Suo*)
Fructus Meliae Toosendanis (*Chuan Lian Zi*)
Caulis Sargentodoxae (*Hong Teng*)
Herba Patriniae Heterophyllae (*Bai Jiang Cao*)
Radix Et Rhizoma Rhei (*Da Huang*)
Radix Dioscoreae Hypoglaucae (*Bi Xie*)
Fructus Liquidambaris Taiwaniae (*Lu Lu Tong*)
Rhizoma Paridis Polyphyllae (*Quan Shen*)

Bao Luo Hua Yu Tang Jia Jian

Radix Sanguisorbae (*Sheng Di Yu*)
Radix Cyathulae (*Chuan Niu Xi*)
stir-fried Squama Manitis (*Shan Jia*)
Semen Vaccariae Segetalis (*Wang Bu Liu Xing*)
Fructus Liquidambaris Taiwaniae (*Lu Lu Tong*)
Semen Citri Reticulatae (*Ju He*)
Rhizoma Curcumae Zedoariae (*E Zhu*)
Radix Angelicae Sinensis (*Dang Gui*)
Caulis Milletiae Seu Spatholobi (*Ji Xue Teng*)
salt-fried Cortex Phellodendri (*Huang Bai*)
Herba Sargassi (*Hai Zao*)
Semen Plantaginis (*Che Qian Zi*)

Zhou Ming-qi *et al.* give this formula in a case history discussion of female infertility[2]. The therapeutic principles given are to course the liver and rectify the qi, quicken the blood and transform stasis, and soften the hard and scatter nodulation while simultaneously clearing damp heat. They also say that Radix Sanguisorbae and Radix Cyathulae resolve the lower burner of all sorts of hot toxins since they attack, scatter, and sweep away filth and turbidity.

Yin Qiao Hong Jiang Jie Du Tang

Flos Lonicerae Japonicae (*Yin Hua*)
Fructus Forsythiae Suspensae (*Lian Qiao*)
Caulis Sargentodoxae (*Hong Teng*)
Herba Patriniae Heterophyllae (*Bai Jiang Cao*)
Cortex Radicis Moutan (*Dan Pi*)
Fructus Gardeniae Jasminoidis (*Sheng Shan Zhi*)
Radix Rubrus Paeoniae Lactiflorae (*Chi Shao*)
Semen Pruni Persicae (*Tao Ren*)
Rhizoma Corydalis Yanhusuo (*Yan Hu Suo*)
Fructus Meliae Toosendanis (*Chuan Lian Zi*)

---

[2] Zhou Ming-qi, *et al.*, "Records of 2 Successful Cases of Female Infertility," *Zhong Yi Za Zhi (Journal of Traditional Chinese Medicine)*, Vol. 33, No. 5, p. 12-13

4

A General Overview of Modern Chinese Fertility Protocols

As mentioned above, in China today, there is a tendency to treat infertility using a combination of TCM pattern discrimination, modern Western disease diagnosis, and a multiphasic prescriptive regime coordinated with the menstrual cycle. Chinese research has shown that TCM herbal therapy is capable of reestablishing the balance of female reproductive hormones throughout the cycle in infertile women with endocrine dyscrasias. In one study, "It was observed that first FSH increased, then the ratio of blood LH to FSH decreased, the blood E_2 (ovarian hormone secretion) level rose, the LH surge occurred, and ovulation and pregnancy occurred."[1] In research on secondary anovulation due to insufficiency of hypothalamus-pituitary function, supplementing the kidneys treatment increased the pituitary's response to LH-RH and resulted in ovulation and pregnancy.

This section begins with a summary of a recent Chinese article which itself summarizes the main Western medical causes of female infertility and the TCM patterns most commonly associated with these. This is followed by a summary of an article on boosting the kidneys in coordination with four other methods in the treatment of infertility. This article is characteristic of modern Chinese approaches to female infertility which emphasize kidney supplementation. Then, in the next

---

[1]   Yu Jin, "Research on Combining Traditional Chinese and Western Medicine in Female Infertility," *Zhong Guo Zhong Xi Yi Jie He Za Zhi (Journal of Integrated Traditional Chinese and [Modern] Western Medicine)*, No. 10, 1987, p. 617

several chapters, follow a number of modern protocols for each of the main Western causes of female infertility. Several of the protocols below address infertility from the point of view of rebalancing endocrine dyscrasias, thus promoting ovulation and correcting any luteal phase defect or deficiency. This is followed by a single protocol addressing midcycle bleeding. Although this is not a cause of infertility, it does involve an endocrine dyscrasia which may be associated with infertility. Next is a protocol for premature ovarian failure due possibly to thyroiditis. Another several protocols address fallopian tube blockage. Then there are a number of protocols for polycystic ovarian syndrome, endometriosis, and antisperm antibodies.

However, before immediately jumping to descriptions of these various protocols, it is important to know that the Chinese journal literature seems to be unanimous concerning the main therapeutic needs during each of the four phases of the cycle. During phase I, emphasis is on recuperating the blood and kidney yin. The menses has just finished and the sea of blood is relatively empty. Therefore, the body is attempting to nourish the blood and enrich yin.

During phase II or ovulation, emphasis is on warming the *jing* and quickening the blood. These principles seem to be based on the rise in basal body temperature right after ovulation and the fact that women with stagnation and stasis experience *mittelschmerz* or lower abdominal, ovulatory pain. It is said that since yin has become relatively replete at this point, it catalyzes the speedy growth of yang. Therapeutically, if yang is insufficient at this stage, it can retard ovulation and lead to stagnation. However, although most of the fertility protocols described below emphasize the need to warm the uterus during ovulation, in some women, yang becomes pathologically replete at this stage. In those cases, heat needs to be cleared from the blood *fen* or level.

During phase III or the premenstruum, the emphasis is on supplementing yang while strengthening the spleen and rectifying the liver as necessary. Supplementation of yang is based on the fact that, if there is a luteal phase defect, the basal body temperature drops too soon. In normally healthy women, both yin and yang are exuberant during this phase.

During phase IV, the emphasis is on quickening the blood, transforming stasis, and balancing the menses. By the end of menstruation yin and yang are both insufficient.

These principles appear to be self-evident. Li Heng-you, whose protocol is described below, relates these four phases and their dominant therapeutic principles to the following TCM continuum:

Phase I	Phase II	Phase III	Phase IV
kidneys	*tian gui*	*chong ren*	uterus

Abnormalities in Basal Body Temperature and Infertility

In the modern Chinese journal literature on female infertility, much interest is paid to the basal body temperature (BBT) as an indication of proper ovarian and corpus luteal function. Researchers in the People's Republic of China are attempting to correlate abnormalities in the BBT with TCM disease mechanisms and their associated patterns. Xia Gui-cheng gives the following account of such correlation in the Shanghai Journal of TCM, October 1992.[2]

Xia identifies six types or categories of BBT anomalies in women suffering from infertility due to an ovarian or luteal phase defect.

---

[2]   Xia Gui-cheng, "Use of the Basal Body Temperature in Pattern Discrimination for Patients with Infertility and Amenorrhea," *Shang Hai Zhong Yi Yao Za Zhi (Shanghai Journal of TCM)*, No. 10, 1992, p. 18-19

Type 1 is characterized by a slow rise in temperature during the hyperthermic or luteal phase. If plotted on a graph, this rise would look like stair steps. Type 2 is characterized by a consistently low BBT throughout the luteal phase. In this case, the BBT only rises 0.2-0.3°C. Type 3 refers to a short hyperthermic phase and is further divided into three subcategories. These are 1) extremely short, a hyperthermic phase lasting only 6-7 days; 2) short, a hyperthermic phase lasting only 8-9 days; and 3) slightly short, a hyperthermic phase lasting only 10-11 days. The hyperthermic phase should last more like 12-13 days. Type 4 is characterized by a slow descent in BBT beginning 3-5 days before the onset of the period instead of dropping precipitously the day before. Type 5 refers to a BBT which first rises, then after 3-5 days descends, and thereafter goes up again. Type 6 is characterized by a BBT during the hyperthermic phase which goes up and down erratically. If plotted on a graph, its "curve" looks like the teeth of a saw.

Xia goes on to correlate types 1, 2, and 3 with an insufficiency of water and fire, or dual vacuity of yin and yang, with yang vacuity predominating. In the case of a short hyperthermic phase, Xia attributes this to simultaneous qi vacuity as well. Types 4 and 5 are categorized as due to insufficiency of yang qi with dual spleen/kidney vacuity. Type 6 Xia correlates in all cases with kidney vacuity complicated, depending upon the case, by loss of harmony with the heart, liver, spleen, and/or stomach. In particular, Xia says type 6 is commonly complicated heart/liver depressive fire.

These observations are corroborated by my own clinical experience. If such correlations are true, patients' monthly BBT charts can help establish their TCM patterns from month to month, thereby helping the practitioner refine their prescriptive methodology. The following tables further clarifies these ideas.

Human Induced Regulation of the Menstrual Cycle, BBT Coordinated with TCM Therapeutic Principles

Phase I: Postmenstruum; Proliferative Stage; Hypothermal Phase

Days 4-9 approximately

BBT Low

Tx principles: Nourish the blood and supplement the kidneys, rectify qi and regulate blood

Goal: Promote follicular development

Phase II: Intermenstruum; Ovulatory Stage; Transitional Phase

Days 10-16 approximately

BBT goes from low to high

Tx principles: Warm yang, move the qi and quicken the blood, open the connecting vessels

Goal: Promote ovulation

Phase III: Premenstruum; Luteal Phase; Secretive Phase; Hyperthermal Phase

Days 17-28 approximately

BBT should stay high until day 26-27

Tx principles: Nourish and warm the kidneys, regulate the blood and rectify qi

Goal: Fortify function of the corpus luteum

Phase IV: Menses

Days 1-5 approximately

BBT low

Tx principles: Move the qi and quicken the blood

Goal: Regulate the menses

Types of BBT Curves Correlated to the Menstrual Cycle

Normal: Biphasic; distinct differentiation between hypothermal and hyperthermal phases
TCM Dx: Kidney *jing* sufficient, yin & yang in harmony, qi & blood disinhibited

Monophasic: Low BBT throughout the month; no hyperthermal phase
TCM Dx: Kidney yang insufficiency

Prolonged Hypothermal Phase: BBT remains low too long
TCM Dx: Primarily kidney yin vacuity; possibly kidney spleen dual vacuity

Prolonged Transition to Hyperthermal Phase: Change from hypo to hyperthermal phases prolonged more than 3 days
TCM Dx: Kidney yang vacuity, liver depression

"Horse-shaped" Hyperthermal Phase: BBT rises, but, after 3-5 days, descends close to low temperature. Then afterwards goes back up again
TCM Dx: Yang qi insufficiency, kidney spleen dual vacuity

Sawtoothed Hyperthermal Phase: BBT goes up and down irregularly
TCM Dx: Yang vacuity with loss of harmony of the heart, liver, spleen, and stomach: commonly liver depression or heart liver depressive fire

Prolonged Transition to Hypothermal Phase: BBT slowly descends 3-5 days before onset of period
TCM Dx: Yang qi insufficiency, kidney spleen dual vacuity

Shortened Hyperthermal Phase: BBT goes down too soon after ovulation
TCM Dx: Kidney spleen yang vacuity
Extremely short: 6-7 days   Short: 8-9 days   Slightly short: 10-11 days

The Main Western Diseases Associated with Female Infertility

Li Xian-yun, writing in the *Shang Hai Zhong Yi Yao Za Zhi (Shanghai Journal of TCM)* in 1992, summarizes the main Western diseases or conditions involved in female infertility.[3] These are listed as fallopian tube blockage, menstrual irregularity (*i.e.*, hormonal dyscrasia and ovarian dysfunction), endometriosis, polycystic ovarian syndrome, and uterine myoma. Li, following Wang Qing-ren's lead in the Qing Dynasty, emphasizes the importance of quickening the blood and transforming stasis in the treatment of infertility. However, he also makes some very interesting comments about the main TCM disease mechanisms at work in each of these conditions.

Fallopian Tube Blockage

Li says that 40% of female infertility is due to fallopian tube blockage which in turn is usually due to either endometriosis or the sequelae of pelvic inflammatory disease. Mostly this condition is treated by quickening the blood and transforming stasis. However, one must distinguish between the following different types of stasis.

1. Qi stagnation, blood stasis

2. Cold damp stasis and stagnation

3. Phlegm dampness stasis and stagnation

4. Qi vacuity, blood stasis

5. Accumulation of heat, stasis and obstruction

---

[3] Li Xian-yun, "The Use of Blood-Activating, Spleen-Transforming in Infertility," *Shang Hai Zhong Yi Yao Za Zhi (Shanghai Journal of TCM)*, No. 4, 1992, p. 22-24

Li says that of 87 women treated for fallopian tube blockage, 75 subsequently conceived, for a success rate of 86.1%. In the case history Li gives, the woman was treated for more than a year before her tubes became open and patent and then was treated for another 3 months to supplement her kidneys and strengthen her spleen before becoming pregnant.

Menstrual Irregularity

Li uses the term menstrual irregularity to cover infertility due to hormonal imbalance and ovarian dysfunction. Li says that 20% of female infertility is due to this cause. He says that basically this condition is due to:

    1. Kidney vacuity, liver depression, and spleen weakness

These 3 basic disease mechanisms are then complicated by:

    2. More pronounced liver depression, qi stagnation

    3. Vacuity cold of the *chong* and *ren*

    4. Blood stasis

The case history Li includes describes 5 months of therapy in order to quicken the blood and transform stasis, warm the *jing* and regulate the menses before the woman conceived. The fact that Li sees kidney vacuity, liver depression, and spleen vacuity as the basic three mechanisms associated with hormonal dyscrasia resulting in subfertility or infertility is born out by my own clinical experience.

Endometriosis

Li says endometriosis accounts for another 30-40% of female infertility. He says that it is due mostly to qi stagnation and blood stasis with blockage and stagnation of the *mai luo*. Li says that of 38 cases treated, 10 conceived after their menses became normal and they had no menstrual pain.

Polycystic Ovarian Syndrome

This condition is characterized by scanty periods or amenorrhea, hirsutism, obesity, and infertility. Li does not give any percentage of how many infertile women suffer from this condition. Li says that to treat this condition, one should primarily quicken the blood and transform stasis while simultaneously supplementing the kidneys. Out of 5 cases mentioned, 4 conceived after Chinese medicinal therapy.

Uterine Myoma

Li says that these are due to essentially three mechanisms:

1. Blood stasis

2. Phlegm dampness

3. Cold congelation

Although these discussions by Li of the various Western diseases associated with female infertility are not necessarily categorically complete, they nevertheless do provide an overview of the modern Chinese methodology of treating female infertility. This methodology is characterized by dual diagnosis. Dual diagnosis means that treatment is given predicated on both a Western disease diagnosis and a TCM pattern diagnosis.

Kidney Supplementation & the Treatment of Female Infertility

Zhang Hui-he and Tu Ding-rong, in an article published in 1992, recommend four sets of therapeutic principles for the treatment of female infertility.[4] All of them include boosting the kidneys. As Zhang and Tu state, the main treatment principles are to nourish the blood and warm the kidneys. However, because female infertility patients' patterns are often complicated phlegm dampness, liver depression, and blood stasis, one cannot rely on those therapeutic principles alone. Therefore, Zhang and Tu give four sets of therapeutic principles for the treatment of infertility. Although Zhang and Tu do not correlate these methods with named TCM patterns, the pathognomonic signs and symptoms of the first method primarily describe a kidney vacuity pattern, the second a liver depression pattern, the third a phlegm dampness pattern, and the fourth a blood stasis pattern.

1. Boost the Kidneys & Quicken the Blood Method

Pathognomonic manifestations: Typically ovarian function is insufficient, ovulation may be hindered, and there may be pathological changes during the endometrial proliferative phase or during the endocrine secretive phase. The menses is typically late and its amount is scant. The color of the blood is dark and dusky. There is dizziness and tinnitus, the essence spirit is exhausted and weary, the low back and knees are sore and weak, sexual desire is diminished, urination is clear and long, the tongue is pale, its coating is white and moist, and the pulse is deep and fine. Also typically, the BBT's hyperthermic phase is unstable and corpus luteal function after ovulation is insufficient.

Rx:

Radix Codonopsis Pilosulae (*Dang Shen*)

---

[4]   Zhong Hui-he and Tu Ding-rong, "*Bu Yun Zheng Cong Shen Bian Zhi Si Fa* (Four Methods for the Differential Treatment of Infertility Through the Kidneys)," *Si Chuan Zhong Yi (Sichuan Traditional Chinese Medicine),* No. 12, 1992, p. 6-7

Radix Astragali Membranacei (*Huang Qi*)
Radix Rehmanniae (*Sheng Di*)
Radix Dioscoreae Oppositae (*Shan Yao*)
Radix Angelicae Sinensis (*Dang Gui*)
Rhizoma Ligustici Wallichii (*Chuan Xiong*)
Radix Dipsaci (*Xu Duan*)
Radix Albus Paeoniae Lactiflorae (*Bai Shao*)
Cortex Eucommiae Ulmoidis (*Du Zhong*)
Semen Cuscutae (*Tu Si Zi*)
Herba Cistanchis (*Rou Cong Rong*)
Placenta Hominis (*Zi He Che*)
mix-fried Radix Glycyrrhizae (*Zhi Gan Cao*)

Administer 5-7 *ji* or *bao*, packets, during the luteal phase.

2. Boost the Kidneys & Course the Liver Method

Pathognomonic manifestations: In this case, the older woman has gone without child for a number of years. Her menstruation may be normal and gynecological examination reveals that her fallopian tubes may be open and unobstructed and her uterine endometrium normal. Hormonal secretions may be slightly low or normal. The rise in BBT temperature may be obviously retarded and the hyperthermal phase typically lasts less than 8-9 days. Premenstrually, there is chest oppression, vexation and agitation, and breast distention and pain. When the period comes, there may be low back soreness and weakness or pain in the legs and feet with tinnitus. After the period, there is scant, white abnormal vaginal discharge and the vagina is dry and astringent with obvious decline in sexual desire.

Rx:

Radix Angelicae Sinensis (*Dang Gui*)
Fructus Trichosanthis Kirlowii (*Gua Lou*)
Rhizoma Cyperi Rotundi (*Xiang Fu*)

Fructus Aesculi (*Su Luo Zi*)
Rhizoma Ligustici Wallichii (*Chuan Xiong*)
Radix Dipsaci (*Xu Duan*)
Cortex Eucommiae Ulmoidis (*Du Zhong*)
Semen Cuscutae (*Tu Si Zi*)
Folium Photinae (*Shi Nan Ye*)
Fructus Akebiae Trifoliatae (*Ba Yue Zha*)
Herba Epimedii (*Xian Ling Pi*)
Herba Cistanchis (*Rou Cong Rong*)
Fructus Lycii Chinensis (*Gou Qi Zi*)

Beginning 3-5 days before the onset of menstruation, give 7-10 *ji* of the above medicinals in unbroken succession.

3. Boost the Kidneys & Disperse Fat Method

Dispersing fat here refers to dispersing phlegm dampness in women who are typically obese.

Pathognomonic manifestations: There is either chronic infertility or a history of miscarriage with 2 years or more since last conceiving. The patient's body is fat and their face is sallow white. There is dizziness, they tend to be lazy or inactive and are not well motivated. They are also frequently drowsy. Their mouth is slimy and they have excessive phlegm. Their chest is oppressed and their abdomen distended. There is a pasty, excessive white vaginal discharge and their menses is usually late, sometimes coming only once every 50-70 days. Its amount is scant or there is amenorrhea. Their tongue is slimy and their pulse is slippery. Many of these women may have uterine myomas or fallopian tube blockage. Their BBT may suggest anovulation.

Rx:

Radix Angelicae Sinensis (*Dang Gui*)

Rhizoma Ligustici Wallichii (*Chuan Xiong*)
prepared Radix Rehmanniae (*Shu Di*)
Radix Morindae Officinalis (*Ba Ji Tian*)
Semen Trigonellae Foeni-greaci (*Hu Lu Ba*)
processed Rhizoma Pinelliae Ternatae (*Ban Xia*)
Tuber Curcumae (*Guang Yu Jin*)
Semen Sinapis Albae (*Bai Jie Zi*)
Massa Medica Fermentata (*Shen Qu*)
Fructus Crataegi (*Shan Zha*)
Rhizoma Arisaematis (*Nan Xing*)
Spina Gleditschiae Chinensis (*Jiao Ci*)

Beginning 5 days after the onset of menstruation, give 7-10 *ji*, or during menstruation give 1 *ji* per day. If there is amenorrhea, it is alright to use progesterone to stimulate menstruation. Then, beginning 3-5 days before the expected onset of menstruation, give 7-10 *ji* in succession.

4. Boost the Kidneys & Dispel Stasis Method

Pathognomonic manifestations: Women requiring these methods commonly suffer from uterine myomas, endometriosis, and fallopian tube blockage. Their menses are irregular, there is dysmenorrhea, excessive abnormal vaginal discharge, and urgent pain in the lower abdomen which worsens as the period draws closer. There is also dizziness and ringing in the ears, the memory is poor, and there is either fear of cold or vexatious heat. The facial complexion is dark and dusky and the tongue has ecchymotic spots or patches or the sublingual veins may be distended.

Rx:

Radix Angelicae Sinensis (*Dang Gui*)
Rhizoma Ligustici Wallichii (*Chuan Xiong*)
Semen Pruni Persicae (*Tao Ren*)

Ramulus Cinnamomi (*Gui Zhi*)
Radix Rubrus Paeoniae Lactiflorae (*Chi Shao*)
Rhizoma Sparganii (*San Leng*)
Rhizoma Curcumae Zedoariae (*E Zhu*)
processed Carapax Amydae (*Bie Jia*)
Concha Haliotidis (*Pao Jia Zhu*)
Radix Linderae Strychnifoliae (*Wu Yao*)
Rhizoma Corydalis Yanhusuo (*Yan Hu Suo*)
Herba Cynomorii Songarici (*Suo Yang*)
Radix Dipsaci (*Xu Duan*)
Cornu Degelatinum Cervi (*Lu Jiao Shuang*)

It is alright to use these medicinals daily even during the menses.

5

Endocrine Dyscrasias: Anovulation, Luteal Phase Defect, Midcycle Bleeding, & Premature Ovarian Failure

Ovulation and successful implantation of the fertilized zygote are controlled by hormones secreted primarily by the pituitary and ovaries. However, thyroid disturbances and adrenal hyperplasia can also affect a woman's endocrine balance and thus ovulation and menstruation. The main hormones involved in female fertility are follicle-stimulating hormone (FSH), luteinizing hormone (LH), various estrogens, and progesterone. We have discussed the physiology of these hormones above in Chapter 2 on modern Western medicine and infertility. The two main endocrine pathologies causing female infertility are anovulation and a luteal phase defect. In the first case, no egg is released which can unite with the male sperm to form a fertilized zygote. In the second, although fertilization may take place, the endometrial lining is shed before the zygote can implant success-fully. In this case, the woman may be conceiving but continuously aborting the conceptus.

Modern TCM links ovarian function to the kidneys and suggests that kidney insufficiency, either congenital or due to age, is a factor in most cases of female infertility having to do with ovarian function. Both modern Western medicine and modern TCM recognize the relationship between the mind and emotions, the hypothalamus, the pituitary and hypophysis, and the ovaries. In TCM, this relationship is largely spoken of in terms of Chinese liver function and the flow of qi. In addition, I believe it is important to take into account the role of intestinal dysbiosis and especially candidiasis in both thyroid and ovarian dysfunction. These may lead to hyperallergic and thence to autoimmune states causing thyroiditis and ovaritis which, in turn, can negatively affect these endocrine glands' hormonal functioning. I discuss this in a separate chapter below. As yet, I have not seen any Chinese discussion of this aspect of endocrine dyscrasia in the *fu ke* literature.

The following summaries of research protocols have been taken mostly from recent Chinese TCM journals with some additions from modern Chinese case history and formula compendium books.

1. Feng Du-xiong's Protocol for Endocrine Dyscrasia Infertility[1]

In this study of the treatment of 110 cases of female infertility dating from 1985, two basic formulas were used. One formula was administered from days 4-14 or from the end of menstruation through ovulation. The other formula was administered from the end of ovulation through at least the beginning of the period. These two formulas were modified with additions and subtractions as necessary. Of the women receiving these two formulas, 43 were diagnosed as suffering from kidney vacuity, 23 from liver depression, and 44 from blood stasis. Both basic formulas attempt to address these three key disease mechanisms.

Rx: Postmenstrual Formula

Sclerotium Poriae Cocoris (*Fu Ling*)
Radix Rehmanniae (*Sheng Di*)

---

[1]   Feng Du-xiong, "Analysis of Success in Treating 110 Cases of Infertility," *Shang Hai Zhong Yi Yao Za Zhi (Shanghai Journal of TCM)*, No. 9, 1985, p. 18-20

Fructus Liquidambaris Taiwaniae (*Lu Lu Tong*)
Flos Caryophylli (*Ding Xiang*)
Ramulus Cinnamomi (*Gui Zhi*)
Radix Achyranthis Bidentatae (*Niu Xi*)
Herba Epimedii (*Xian Ling Pi*)
Rhizoma Polygonati (*Huang Jing*)
prepared Radix Rehmanniae (*Shu Di*)
Squama Manitis (*Chuan Shan Jia*)
Folium Photiniae Serrulatae Seu Piperis Wallichii (*Shi Nan Ye*)

Ovulatory Formula

Sclerotium Poriae Cocoris (*Fu Ling*)
Folium Photiniae Serrulatae Seu Piperis Wallichii (*Shi Nan Ye*)
Rhizoma Cibotii Barometsis (*Gou Ji*)
Semen Trigonellae Foeni-graeci (*Hu Lu Ba*)
Radix Rehmanniae (*Sheng Di*)
prepared Radix Rehmanniae (*Shu Di*)
Fluoritum (*Zi Shi Ying*)
Herba Epimedii (*Xian Ling Pi*)
Herba Cistanchis (*Rou Cong Rong*)
Fructus Ligustri Lucidi (*Nu Zhen Zi*)
Herba Curculiginis Orchoidis (*Xian Mao*)
Cornu Degelatinum Cervi (*Lu Jiao Shuang*)

If one analyzes the ingredients of these two formulas, one can see that from the end of menstruation through ovulation the intent is to supplement the liver and kidneys, warm the *jing*, quicken the blood and transform stasis. Whereas, the intent of the postovulatory formula is primarily focused on strengthening yang.

Folium Photiniae Serrulatae is an uncommon medicinal in general practice. It is acrid, bitter, and neutral, enters the liver and kidneys, expels wind, opens the *luo*, and boosts the kidneys. It treats female infertility with chilly low back and menstrual irregularity.

No overall success rates are given in this study. Therapy stretched from 1-24 months with an average of 5.8 months per patient. For women below 30 years of age, the average duration of therapy was 5.1 months. For women over 40, the average duration was 13 months. One thing these numbers suggest is that the older the woman, the longer she should expect TCM therapy for infertility to take before it is effective.

2. Xu Jiang-sheng's Protocol for Endocrine Dyscrasia Infertility[2]

This protocol from 1988 aims at regulating the female hormones during different stages of the menstrual cycle, to stimulate ovulation, and promote fertility. In this protocol, there is a different set of therapeutic principles and formula for each of the four phases.

Phase I, postmenstruation, proliferative phase, days 4-10

During this phase, the follicles develop, estrogen gradually increases, and the endometrial lining begins to proliferate. In terms of TCM theory, yin is growing and blood is being replaced.

Therapeutic principles: Supplement the kidneys, store essence, and enrich yin

Rx: Follicle-stimulating Formula

Placenta Hominis (*Zi He Che*)
Rhizoma Curculiginis Orchoidis (*Xian Mao*)
Herba Epimedii (*Xian Ling Pi*)

---

[2] Xu Jiang-sheng, "Understanding the Methods of Regulating the Menstrual Cycle Using TCM," *Shang Hai Zhong Yi Yao Za Zhi (Shanghai Journal of TCM)*, No. 3, 1988, p. 10-12

Semen Cuscutae (*Tu Si Zi*)
Radix Dioscoreae Oppositae (*Shan Yao*)
Radix Polygoni Multiflori (*He Shou Wu*)
Radix Angelicae Sinensis (*Dang Gui*)
Fructus Ligustri Lucidi (*Nu Zhen Zi*)
Radix Dipsaci (*Xu Duan*)
prepared Radix Rehmanniae (*Shu Di*)
Fructus Lycii Chinensis (*Gou Qi*)

Phase II, midcyle, ovulation, days 11-14

During this phase, the follicles reach maturation. The secretion of estrogen reaches its peak and this stimulates the pituitary to secrete large amounts of LH. This induces the mature follicle to rupture and complete ovulation. In terms of TCM theory, yin which is replete transforms into yang. As Xu states, "This concept is the key to inducing (an) artificially (normal) menstrual cycle through the use of Ovulation-stimulating Formula."

Therapeutic principles: Supplement the kidneys and stimulate ovulation

Rx: Ovulation-stimulating Formula

Rhizoma Curculiginis Orchoidis (*Xian Mao*)
Rhizoma Ligustici Wallichii (*Chuan Xiong*)
Herba Lycopi Lucidi (*Ze Lan*)
Herba Epimedii (*Xian Ling Pi*)
Semen Leonuri Heterophylli (*Chong Wei Zi*)
Radix Achyranthis Bidentatae (*Niu Xi*)
Radix Rubrus Paeoniae Lactiflorae (*Chi Shao*)
Flos Carthami Tinctorii (*Hong Hua*)
Fructus Liquidambaris Taiwaniae (*Lu Lu Tong*)
Radix Angelicae Sinensis (*Dang Gui*)
Rhizoma Cyperi Rotundi (*Xiang Fu*)
Semen Vaccariae Segetalis (*Wang Bu Liu Xing*)

Phase III, premenstruum, secretion phase, days 14-28

This phase runs from ovulation to the onset of the period. During this time, the corpus luteum reaches maturity. It maintains progesterone production until degeneration and this progesterone increases the endometrial thickening. In terms of TCM theory, during this phase yin is full and yang is growing, the uterus is warm and is waiting for conception.

Therapeutic principles: Supplement the kidneys and warm yang, boost the qi and nourish the blood

Rx: Corpus Luteum-stimulating Formula

prepared Radix Rehmanniae (*Shu Di*)
Radix Angelicae Sinensis (*Dang Gui*)
Radix Dioscoreae Oppositae (*Shan Yao*)
Herba Epimedii (*Xian Ling Pi*)
Herba Cistanchis (*Rou Cong Rong*)
Radix Codonopsis Pilosulae (*Dang Shen*)
Rhizoma Curculiginis Orchoidis (*Xian Mao*)
Semen Cuscutae (*Tu Si Zi*)
Radix Glycyrrhizae (*Gan Cao*)
Cortex Cinnamomi (*Rou Gui*)
Fructus Rubi (*Fu Pen Zi*)

Phase IV, menstruation, days 1-4

This phase corresponds to the onset of menstruation. The endometrial lining is sloughed and there is a bloody discharge from the vagina. Attending this there is a rapid drop in female hormones, both estrogen and progesterone. TCM theory explains this thus: Yang becomes heavy and strong and is transformed into yin. This is based on the *I Ching* concept that yang when extreme transforms into yin. The sea of blood becomes full. In response to plummeting kidney yang which has been transformed into yin and a consequent relative vacuity of kidney qi to astringe the lower yin or vaginal meatus, blood is thence discharged in the form of the menstrual flow. This corresponds to the drop in BBT the day before the onset of menstruation.

Therapeutic principles: (If the menses is not normal,) move the qi and quicken the blood

Rx: Menstruation-regulating Formula

Radix Angelicae Sinensis (*Dang Gui*)
Semen Pruni Persicae (*Tao Ren*)
Herba Lycopi Lucidi (*Ze Lan*)
Radix Rubrus Paeoniae Lactiflorae (*Chi Shao*)
Flos Carthami Tinctorii (*Hong Hua*)
Radix Achyranthis Bidentatae (*Niu Xi*)
Rhizoma Ligustici Wallichii (*Chuan Xiong*)
Rhizoma Cyperi Rotundi (*Xiang Fu*)
Herba Leonuri Heterophylli (*Yi Mu Cao*)
prepared Radix Rehmanniae (*Shu Di*)
Pericarpium Viridis Citri Reticulatae (*Qing Pi*)
Pericarpium Citri Reticulatae (*Chen Pi*)

All the above formulas are to be modified according to the presenting signs and symptoms of each patient. No success rates are given by Tang.

3. Yung Wen-lan's Protocol for Endocrine Dyscrasia Infertility[3]

Like the above, this protocol from 1987 uses a four phase division. Of the 132 cases treated in this research, 79.5% were diagnosed with kidney yang vacuity and 20.5% with kidney yin vacuity. That means the author identified some element of kidney vacuity in every case.

Phase I

Therapeutic principles: Supplement the liver and kidneys, nourish the blood and regulate the menses

Rx: *Liu Wei Di Huang Wan Jia Jian*

prepared Radix Rehmanniae (*Shu Di*)
Radix Glycyrrhizae (*Gan Cao*)
Fructus Corni Officinalis (*Shan Zhu Yu*)
Radix Albus Paeoniae Lactiflorae (*Bai Shao*)
Radix Dioscoreae Oppositae (*Shan Yao*)
Radix Pseudostellariae (*Tai Zi Shen*)
Radix Angelicae Sinensis (*Dang Gui*)
Gelatinum Plastri Testudinis (*Gui Ban Jiao*)
Semen Cuscutae (*Tu Si Zi*)
Fructus Lycii Chinensis (*Gou Qi Zi*)
Cortex Radicis Moutan (*Dan Pi*)
Sclerotium Poriae Cocoris (*Fu Ling*)

---

[3] Yung Wan-lan, "Clinical Observations in Treating 132 Cases of Primary Infertility with Chinese Herbs (Induced) Artificial Cycle," *Shang Hai Zhong Yi Yao Za Zhi (Shanghai Journal of TCM)*, No. 6, 1987, p. 18-19

Phase II

Therapeutic principles: Supplement the kidneys and boost the qi, warm the *jing* and quicken the blood

Rx:

prepared Radix Rehmanniae (*Shu Di*)
Sclerotium Poriae Cocoris (*Fu Ling*)
mix-fried Radix Glycyrrhizae (*Zhi Gan Cao*)
Radix Angelicae Sinensis (*Dang Gui*)
Radix Salviae Miltiorrhizae (*Dan Shen*)
Herba Epimedii (*Xian Ling Pi*)
Herba Lycopi Lucidi (*Ze Lan*)
Rhizoma Curculiginis Orchoidis (*Xian Mao*)
Semen Cuscutae (*Tu Si Zi*)
Rhizoma Cyperi Rotundi (*Xiang Fu*)
Semen Pruni Persicae (*Tao Ren*)
Radix Codonopsis Pilosulae (*Dang Shen*)

Phase III

Therapeutic principles: Warm the kidneys and supplement the spleen

Rx:

Radix Angelicae Sinensis (*Dang Gui*)
prepared Radix Rehmanniae (*Shu Di*)
Semen Cuscutae (*Tu Si Zi*)
Fructus Lycii Chinensis (*Gou Qi*)
Sclerotium Poriae Cocoris (*Fu Ling*)
Radix Codonopsis Pilosulae (*Dang Shen*)
Radix Morindae Officinalis (*Ba Ji Tian*)
mix-fried Radix Glycyrrhizae (*Zhi Gan Cao*)
Radix Dioscoreae Oppositae (*Shan Yao*)

117

Herba Epimedii (*Xian Ling Pi*)
Gelatinum Cornu Cervi (*Lu Jiao Jiao*) or
Cornu Degelatinum Cervi (*Lu Jiao Shuang*)

Phase IV

Therapeutic principles: Quicken the blood and regulate the menses

Rx:

Radix Angelicae Sinensis (*Dang Gui*)
Radix Salviae Miltiorrhizae (*Dan Shen*)
Radix Glycyrrhizae (*Gan Cao*)
Rhizoma Ligustici Wallichii (*Chuan Xiong*)
Herba Lycopi Lucidi (*Ze Lan*)
Rhizoma Cyperi Rotundi (*Xiang Fu*)
Sclerotium Poriae Cocoris (*Fu Ling*)
Herba Leonuri Heterophylli (*Yi Mu Cao*)
Radix Rubrus Paeoniae Lactiflorae (*Chi Shao*)

All of the above formulas are to be modified with additions and subtractions as necessary. Seventy-eight point eight percent of the total of 132 cases conceived. Eighty-nine percent of the 27 cases of kidney yin vacuity conceived. While 76.2% of the 105 kidney yang vacuity cases conceived. Tang does not report the average number of cycles treated.

4. Guo Yan-wan's Protocol for Endocrine Dyscrasia Infertility[4]

In this study, the emphasis is on supplementing the *chong* and *ren*, nourishing the blood, regulating the menses, supplementing the heart and spleen, and benefitting the source of blood production. It uses a single formula which is then modified throughout the four phases of the menstrual cycle.

Rx: *Tiao Chong Ren Yang Xue Tang*

prepared Radix Rehmanniae (*Shu Di*)
Semen Cuscutae (*Tu Si Zi*)
mix-fried Radix Glycyrrhizae (*Zhi Gan Cao*)
Radix Dioscoreae Oppositae (*Shan Yao*)
Stamen Nelumbinis Nuciferae (*Lian Xu*)
Sclerotium Poriae Cocoris (*Fu Ling*)
Ramus Loranthis Seu Visci (*Sang Ji Sheng*)
Fructus Lycii Chinensis (*Gou Qi*)
Semen Biotae Orientalis (*Bai Zi Ren*)
Arillus Euphoriae Longanae (*Yuan Rou*) or
Fructus Zizyphi Jujubae (*Da Zao*)

Phase I

Therapeutic principles: Nourish the blood and supplement the *chong* and *ren*

Add the following medicinals:

Radix Codonopsis Pilosulae (*Dang Shen*)

---

[4] Guo Yan-wan, "Conclusions on the Blood Nourishing Formula that Cured 50 Infertility Cases," *Guangzhou TCM College Newspaper*, n.i., n.d.

119

Gelatinum Corii Asini (*E Jiao*)
Fructus Rubi (*Fu Pen Zi*)
Caulis Photinae Serrulatae (*Shi Nan Teng*)

Phase II

Therapeutic principles: Quicken the blood and boost the qi, open the portals and promote the maturation of follicles

Add the following medicinals:

Radix Salviae Miltiorrhizae (*Dan Shen*)
Rhizoma Cyperi Rotundi (*Xiang Fu*)
Radix Astragali Membranacei (*Huang Qi*)
Rhizoma Acori Graminei (*Shi Chang Pu*)

Phase III

Therapeutic principles: Nourish the *chong* and *ren*, course the liver and resolve depression

Make the following modifications:

delete Arillus Euphoriae Longanae or
Fructus Zizyphi Jujubae, and add
Flos Rosae Chinensis (*Yue Ji Hua*)
Rhizoma Polygonati Odorati (*Yu Zhu*).

Phase IV

Add and subtract depending upon the patient's condition during menstruation.

In his discussion of this protocol, Guo makes several observations. First, the kidneys govern reproduction and rule the *chong* and *ren*. Secondly, TCM theory says that in the treatment of infertility one should first regulate menstruation. Third, most infertile women have emotional problems caused by liver qi. If this transforms into fire, it can dry yin and lead to liver/kidney vacuity. Therefore, for coursing the liver and rectifying the qi in infertility, it is best to use flower medicinals, presumably such as Flos Rosae Rugosae (*Mei Gui Hua*), Flos Rosae Chinensis (*Yue Ji Hua*), and Flos Albizziae Julibrissinis (*He Huan Hua*). Fourth, a cold uterus may result from spleen/kidney vacuity. Therefore, care should be taken not to use bitter, cold, heat-clearing medicinals. Neither should one use yang-supplementing medicinals which can dry yin. Caulis Photinae Serrulatae effectively warms the uterus without drying yin. Fifth, infertility due to phlegm dampness is best treated when combined with ingredients to nourish blood and supplement the *chong* and *ren*. And sixth, during ovulation, correct treatment should be based on supplementing the *chong* and *ren* at the same time as quickening the blood and dispelling stasis.

5. Li Heng-you's Protocol for Anovulation[5]

In this protocol, the assumption is made that anovulatory infertility relates to kidney vacuity and that supplementing the kidneys is an indispensable part of treating this condition. It too relies on a multi-phasic approach but unlike the above protocols, it employs three different treatment plans depending upon *bian zheng* diagnosis.

---

[5] Li Heng-you, *Zhong Guo Xian Dai Ming Zhong Yi Yi An Jing Hua (Quintessential Case Histories from Famous Modern Chinese TCM Doctors)*, edited by Zhong Jian Hua *et al.*, Beijing Press, Beijing, 1990, reprinted in *Fleshing Out the Bones*, translated by Charles Chace, Blue Poppy Press, Boulder, CO, 1992, p. 159-169

Kidney Vacuity

In this treatment plan, supplementation of kidney vacuity is the primary therapeutic principle.

Phase I

Therapeutic principles: Supplement the *chong* and *ren* to assist ovulatory function

Rx: *Wu Yao Tiao Jing Wan* plus *Tai Ban Pian*

These are two patent medicines. The second is made from Placenta Hominis (*Zi He Che*). I have not been able to find the ingredients in the first formula.

Phase II

Therapeutic principles: Supplement the kidneys to promote follicular development

Rx: *Zu Rong He Ji*

Semen Cuscutae (*Tu Si Zi*)
Radix Dioscoreae Oppositae (*Shan Yao*)
prepared Radix Rehmanniae (*Shu Di*)
Fructus Lycii Chinensis (*Gou Qi*)
Radix Dipsaci (*Xu Duan*)
Radix Angelicae Sinensis (*Dang Gui*)
Rhizoma Cyperi Rotundi (*Xiang Fu*)
Herba Cistanchis (*Rou Cong Rong*)
Herba Epimedii (*Xian Ling Pi*)

Additions & subtractions based on pattern discrimination: If yin vacuity is pronounced, add Fructus Ligustri Lucidi (*Nu Zhen Zi*) and Herba

Ecliptae Prostratae (*Han Lian Cao*). If yang vacuity is pronounced, add Cornu Degelatinum Cervi (*Lu Jiao Shuang*).

Phase III & IV

Therapeutic principles: Quicken the blood and regulate the menses to promote the arrival of the menses

Rx: *Tiao Jing Huo Xue He Ji*

Radix Angelicae Sinensis (*Dang Gui*)
Semen Cuscutae (*Tu Si Zi*)
Radix Rubrus Paeoniae Lactiflorae (*Chi Shao*)
Herba Lycopi Lucidi (*Ze Lan*)
Sclerotium Poriae Cocoris (*Fu Ling*)
Rhizoma Ligustici Wallichii (*Chuan Xiong*)
Rhizoma Cyperi Rotundi (*Xiang Fu*)

Additions & subtractions based on pattern discrimination: If there is extreme abdominal pain, add: Rhizoma Corydalis Yanhusuo (*Yan Hu*) and Feces Trogopterori Seu Pteromi (*Wu Ling Zhi*). Only add after the menses has begun, not premenstrually. If there is vacuity cold, use *Wen Jing Tang* during the menses.

Rx: *Wen Jing Tang*

Radix Angelicae Sinensis (*Dang Gui*)
Radix Albus Paeoniae Lactiflorae (*Bai Shao*)
Fructus Evodiae Rutecarpae (*Wu Zhu Yu*)
Ramulus Cinnamomi (*Gui Zhi*)
Rhizoma Ligustici Wallichii (*Chuan Xiong*)
Gelatinum Corii Asini (*E Jiao*)
Tuber Ophiopogonis Japonicae (*Mai Dong*)
Cortex Radicis Moutan (*Dan Pi*)
Radix Panacis Ginseng (*Ren Shen*)

Rhizoma Pinelliae Ternatae (*Ban Xia*)
fresh Rhizoma Zingiberis (*Sheng Jiang*)
Radix Glycyrrhizae (*Gan Cao*)

Blood Stasis

In this protocol, supplementation of the kidneys is combined with quickening of the blood and dispelling of stasis.

Phase I

Therapeutic principles: Supplement the kidneys and nourish the *chong* and *ren* to promote follicular development and ovulation

Rx: *Cu Luan Bao Tang*

Radix Dioscoreae Oppositae (*Shan Yao*)
prepared Radix Rehmanniae (*Shu Di*)
Radix Polygoni Multiflori (*He Shou Wu*)
Semen Cuscutae (*Tu Si Zi*)
Radix Angelicae Sinensis (*Dang Gui*)
Herba Cistanchis (*Rou Cong Rong*)

Additions & subtractions based on pattern discrimination: If yang vacuity is pronounced, add Herba Epimedii (*Xian Ling Pi*) and Rhizoma Curculiginis Orchoidis (*Xian Mao*). If yin vacuity is pronounced, add Fructus Ligustri Lucidi (*Nu Zhen Zi*).

Phase II

Therapeutic principles: Quicken the blood and transform stasis to promote maturation and ejection of the ovum

Rx: *Pai Luan Tang*

Radix Angelicae Sinensis (*Dang Gui*)
Radix Rubrus Paeoniae Lactiflorae (*Chi Shao*)
Herba Lycopi Lucidi (*Ze Lan*)
prepared Radix Rehmanniae (*Shu Di*)
Rhizoma Ligustici Wallichii (*Chuan Xiong*)
Semen Pruni Persicae (*Tao Ren*)
Flos Carthami Tinctorii (*Hong Hua*)
Rhizoma Cyperi Rotundi (*Xiang Fu*)

Additions & subtractions based on pattern discrimination: If yang vacuity is pronounced, add Ramulus Cinnamomi (*Gui Zhi*) and Caulis Millettiae Seu Spatholobi (*Ji Xue Teng*). If yin vacuity is pronounced, add Radix Salviae Miltiorrhizae (*Dan Shen*) and Fructus Lycii Chinensis (*Gou Qi Zi*).

Phase III

Therapeutic principles: Regulate the liver and kidneys and nourish the *chong* and *ren* to strengthen the corpus luteum and create a favorable condition for the ovum to implant

Rx: *Ti Huang Di Tang*

Radix Dioscoreae Oppositae (*Shan Yao*)
prepared Radix Rehmanniae (*Shu Di*)
Radix Polygoni Multiflori (*He Shou Wu*)
Radix Dipsaci (*Xu Duan*)
Gelatinum Corii Asini (*E Jiao*)
Plastrum Testudinis (*Gui Ban*)
Fructus Lycii Chinensis (*Gou Qi Zi*)
Herba Cistanchis (*Rou Cong Rong*)

Additions & subtractions based on pattern discrimination: If yang vacuity is more pronounced, add Semen Cuscutae (*Tu Si Zi*) and Radix Angelicae Sinensis (*Dang Gui*). If yin vacuity is more pronounced, add Fructus Ligustri Lucidi (*Nu Zhen Zi*), Radix Salviae Miltiorrhizae (*Dan Shen*), and Herba Ecliptae Prostratae (*Han Lian Cao*).

Phase IV

Therapeutic principles: Quicken the blood and regulate the menses to promote expulsion of the necrotic endometrium and the onset of menstruation. In this protocol, this formula is actually begun day 25, before the actual onset of the period

Rx: *Tiao Jing Huo Xue He Ji* (see above)

Additions & subtractions based on pattern discrimination: If yang vacuity is pronounced, add Caulis Millettiae Seu Spatholobi (*Ji Xue Teng*) and Ramulus Cinnamomi (*Gui Zhi*). If yin vacuity is more pronounced, add Radix Salviae Miltiorrhizae (*Dan Shen*).

Cold Uterus

In this treatment plan, supplementing the kidneys is combined with warming the *jing*. It is used for vacuity cold/ cold uterus.

Phase I

Therapeutic principles: Supplement the spleen and kidneys and nourish the *chong* and *ren* to create the conditions necessary for ovulation

Rx: *Gui Pi Wan* plus *Tai Ban Pian*

Radix Panacis Ginseng (*Ren Shen*)
Radix Astragali Membranacei (*Huang Qi*)
Radix Angelicae Sinensis (*Dang Gui*)

Arillus Euphoriae Longanae (*Long Yan Rou*)
Rhizoma Atractylodis Macrocephalae (*Bai Zhu*)
Radix Saussureae Seu Vladimiriae (*Mu Xiang*)
Sclerotium Poriae Cocoris (*Fu Ling*)
Radix Polygalae Tenuifoliae (*Yuan Zhi*)
Semen Zizyphi Spinosae (*Zao Ren*)
mix-fried Radix Glycyrrhizae (*Zhi Cao*)
fresh Rhizoma Zingiberis (*Sheng Jiang*)
Fructus Zizyphi Jujubae (*Da Zao*)
Placenta Hominis (*Zi He Che*)

Phase II

Therapeutic principles: Warm the kidneys and uterus to promote ovulation

Rx: *Wen Shen Nuan Gong He Ji*

prepared Radix Rehmanniae (*Shu Di*)
Radix Angelicae Sinensis (*Dang Gui*)
Radix Albus Paeoniae Lactiflorae (*Bai Shao*)
Ramus Loranthi Seu Visci (*Sang Ji Sheng*)
Radix Dipsaci (*Xu Duan*)
Herba Cistanchis (*Rou Cong Rong*)
Rhizoma Ligustici Wallichii (*Chuan Xiong*)
Cortex Eucommiae Ulmoidis (*Du Zhong*)
stir-fried Folium Artemesiae Argyii (*Ai Ye*)
Ramulus Cinnamomi (*Gui Zhi*)
Radix Achyranthis Bidentatae (*Niu Xi*)
Semen Alpiniae Katsumadai (*Cao Dou Kou*)

Phases III & IV (days 23 through the period)

Therapeutic principles: Quicken the blood and regulate the menses to promote the onset of the menses

Rx: *Tiao Jing Huo Xue He Ji* (see above) plus

Ramulus Cinnamomi (*Gui Zhi*)
Caulis Millettiae Seu Spatholobi (*Ji Xue Teng*)

All these formulas should be modified according to the patient's presenting pattern, signs, and symptoms. For instance, if there is kidney yang vacuity with liver depression, one should use the first protocol with the addition of medicinals such as Fructus Meliae Toosendanis (*Chuan Lian Zi*), Cortex Albizziae Julibrissinis (*He Huan Pi*), and Radix Achyranthis Bidentatae (*Niu Xi*). One might also alternate protocol 1 with *Xiao Yao San* or *Kai Yu Zhong Yu Tang*. Kidney vacuity is assumed in every one of these three protocols.

6. Sun Ning-quan's Protocol for Luteal Phase Defect[6]

This treatment plan described in a journal article from 1992 focuses on correcting a luteal phase defect in women with a progesterone deficiency. However, analyzing its formulas, it is also effective for promoting ovulation and regulating the menses. Although the title of the journal article from which this protocol is taken mentions specifically luteal phase defect, it regulates reproductive endocrine dyscrasia in general.

Like the above protocols, this treatment plan also assumes that the infertile woman with endocrine dyscrasia suffers from kidney vacuity no matter what other disease mechanisms may also be at work. Sun gives the diagnostic criteria for differentiating the patient's main pattern in his research.

---

[6] Lian Fang, "TCM Treatment of Luteal Phase Defect, An Analysis of 60 Cases," *The Journal of Chinese Medicine*, UK, No. 38, Jan. 1992, p. 19-21

Kidney yin vacuity

Early or late periods with scant blood and no clots, thin vaginal discharge, a red tongue with scant coating, and a deep, thready pulse

Kidney yang vacuity

Late menarche, delayed period, scant, light colored blood, sexual hypoesthesia, low back and knee soreness and weakness, a pale tongue with white coating, and a deep, slow pulse

Spleen/kidney dual vacuity

Menorrhagia, pink in color, no clots, profuse, thin vaginal discharge, fatigue, lack of strength, poor appetite, loose stools, a pale tongue with thin, white coating, and a deep, weak pulse

Kidney vacuity, liver depression

Delayed or irregular menses, profuse or scanty, dark blood with small clots, premenstrual breast distention and pain, low back pain, distention and pain in the lower abdomen during the period, profuse vaginal discharge which may be either thick or thin, a pale tongue with thin, white coating, and a wiry pulse

Phase I

Therapeutic principles: Supplement the kidneys, rectify the qi, and harmonize the blood

Rx:

Fructus Ligustri Lucidi (*Nu Zhen Zi*)
Herba Ecliptae Prostratae (*Han Lian Cao*)
Radix Angelicae Sinensis (*Dang Gui*)

Radix Salviae Miltiorrhizae (*Dan Shen*)
Rhizoma Cyperi Rotundi (*Xiang Fu*)
Radix Saussureae Seu Vladimiriae (*Mu Xiang*)
Radix Linderae Strychnifoliae (*Wu Yao*)
Rhizoma Alismatis (*Ze Xie*)

Additions & subtractions based on pattern discrimination: If there is kidney yin vacuity, add prepared Radix Rehmanniae (*Shu Di*), Radix Pseudostellariae (*Tai Zi Shen*), and Fructus Lycii Chinensis (*Gou Qi Zi*). If there is kidney yang vacuity, add Placenta Hominis (*Zi He Che*), Herba Epimedii (*Xian Ling Pi*), and Herba Cistanchis (*Rou Cong Rong*). If there is spleen vacuity, add Radix Astragali Membranacei (*Huang Qi*), Radix Codonopsis Pilosulae (*Dang Shen*), and Rhizoma Atractylodis Macrocephalae (*Bai Zhu*). If there is kidney vacuity and liver depression, add Radix Bupleuri (*Chai Hu*), Tuber Curcumae (*Yu Jin*), and Radix Albus Paeoniae Lactiflorae (*Bai Shao*).

Phase II

Therapeutic principles: Warm yang and promote the flow of qi and blood in the channels

Rx:

Ramulus Cinnamomi (*Gui Zhi*)
Flos Carthami Tinctorii (*Hong Hua*)
Radix Angelicae Sinensis (*Dang Gui*)
Radix Salviae Miltiorrhizae (*Dan Shen*)
Rhizoma Cyperi Rotundi (*Xiang Fu*)
Radix Saussureae Seu Vladimiriae (*Mu Xiang*)
Radix Linderae Strychnifoliae (*Wu Yao*)
Rhizoma Alismatis (*Ze Xie*)

Additions & subtractions based on pattern discrimination: If there is kidney yin vacuity, add Fructus Ligustri Lucidi (*Nu Zhen Zi*) and

Herba Ecliptae Prostratae (*Han Lian Cao*). If there is kidney yang vacuity, add Cornu Parvum Cervi (*Lu Rong*) and Herba Epimedii (*Xian Ling Pi*). If there is kidney/spleen dual vacuity, add Fructus Citri Sacrodactyli (*Fo Shou*) and Rhizoma Dioscoreae Hypoglaucae (*Bi Xie*). If there is kidney vacuity and liver depression, add Fructus Meliae Toosendanis (*Chuan Lian Zi*) and Tuber Curcumae (*Yu Jin*).

Phase III

Therapeutic principles: Nourish and warm the kidneys, rectify the flow of qi and blood

Rx:

Herba Epimedii (*Xian Ling Pi*)
Rhizoma Curculiginis Orchoidis (*Xian Mao*)
Fructus Ligustri Lucidi (*Nu Zhen Zi*)
Herba Ecliptae Prostratae (*Han Lian Cao*)
Radix Angelicae Sinensis (*Dang Gui*)
Radix Salviae Miltiorrhizae (*Dan Shen*)
Rhizoma Cyperi Rotundi (*Xiang Fu*)
Radix Saussureae Seu Vladimiriae (*Mu Xiang*)
Radix Linderae Strychnifoliae (*Wu Yao*)
Rhizoma Alismatis (*Ze Xie*)

Additions & subtractions based on pattern discrimination: If there is kidney yin vacuity, add prepared Radix Rehmanniae (*Shu Di*), Radix Rehmanniae (*Sheng Di*), Plastrum Testudinis (*Gui Ban*), and Fructus Lycii Chinensis (*Gou Qi*). If there is kidney yang vacuity, add Placenta Hominis (*Zi He Che*), Radix Morindae Officinalis (*Ba Ji Tian*), and Herba Cistanchis (*Rou Cong Rong*). If there is spleen/kidney dual vacuity, add Radix Astragali Membranacei (*Huang Qi*), Radix Codonopsis Pilosulae (*Dang Shen*), and Rhizoma Atractylodis Macrocephalae (*Bai Zhu*). If there is kidney vacuity and liver

131

depression, add Fructus Meliae Toosendanis (*Chuan Lian Zi*) and Radix Bupleuri (*Chai Hu*).

Phase IV

Therapeutic principles: Promote the flow of qi and blood and regulate the menses

Rx:

Semen Pruni Persicae (*Tao Ren*)
Caulis Perillae Frutescentis (*Su Geng*)
Radix Angelicae Sinensis (*Dang Gui*)
Radix Codonopsis Pilosulae (*Dang Shen*)
Rhizoma Cyperi Rotundi (*Xiang Fu*)
Radix Saussureae Seu Vladimiriae (*Mu Xiang*)
Radix Linderae Strychnifoliae (*Wu Yao*)
Rhizoma Alismatis (*Ze Xie*)

Additions & subtractions based on pattern discrimination: If there is kidney yin vacuity, add Fructus Ligustri Lucidi (*Nu Zhen Zi*), Herba Ecliptae Prostratae (*Han Lian Cao*), and Radix Rubrus Paeoniae Lactiflorae (*Chi Shao*). If there is kidney yang vacuity, add Cortex Cinnamomi (*Rou Gui*), Ramulus Cinnamomi (*Gui Zhi*), Radix Puerariae Lobatae (*Ge Geng*), and Fructus Evodiae Rutecarpae (*Wu Zhu Yu*). If there is spleen/kidney dual vacuity, add Pericarpium Citri Reticulatae (*Chen Pi*), Semen Coicis Lachryma-jobi (*Yi Yi Ren*), and Sclerotium Poriae Cocoris (*Fu Ling*). If there is kidney vacuity and liver depression, add Fructus Meliae Toosendanis (*Chuan Lian Zi*), Cortex Radicis Moutan (*Dan Pi*), Rhizoma Corydalis Yanhusuo (*Yuan Hu*), and Radix Rubrus Paeoniae Lactiflorae (*Chi Shao*).

This protocol follows the basic outline of the others above. It assumes the necessity of supplementing the kidneys in all cases of luteal phase defect, nourishes yin postmenstrually, warms the *jing* and quickens the blood at ovulation, warms the kidneys and rectifies the qi premenstrually, and quickens the blood and transforms stasis during menstruation. However, it contains a number of grace notes, such as the addition of Rhizoma Alismatis to keep the kidney yang supplement medicinals from inflaming the *ming men* and Radix Puerariae during phase IV to keep the acrid, warm medicinals for supplementing yang from exhausting the yin of the stomach. Radix Puerariae not only raises yang and generates fluids, it also relaxes the sinews of the shoulders and neck. Up-flushing yang commonly complicates yang vacuity causing upward counterflow of the *du mai*. This counterflowing yang qi spills over into the foot *tai yang* and typically results in stiff shoulders and neck. Radix Puerariae helps to relieve this condition. The theory behind its use is quite profound.

This protocol also suggests a number of other modifications for abnormalities in the menstrual cycle. These modifications help clarify the most typical mechanisms behind certain pathological occurrences commonly encountered in clinical practice.

If there is midcycle bleeding due to liver heat affecting the blood, clear heat from the blood and stop bleeding by adding:

Radix Rehmanniae (*Sheng Di*)
Radix Salviae Miltiorrhizae (*Dan Shen*)
Cortex Radicis Moutan (*Dan Pi*)
Gelatinum Corii Asini (*E Jiao*)

If there is premenstrual spotting, increase the dosages of the kidney warming medicinals and add qi boosters:

Radix Astragali Membranacei (*Huang Qi*)
Radix Codonopsis Pilosulae (*Dang Shen*)
Rhizoma Atractylodis Macrocephalae (*Bai Zhu*)
Rhizoma Cimicifugae (*Sheng Ma*)
Gelatinum Corii Asini (*E Jiao*)

If the period dribbles on for more than 7 days with spotting of dark blood due to stasis, quicken the blood, transform stasis, and stop bleeding by adding:

carbonized Radix Angelicae Sinensis (*Dang Gui*)
carbonized Cacumen Biotae Orientalis (*Ce Bai Ye*)
carbonized Nodus Nelumbinis Nuciferae (*Ou Jie*)

If the period flows too long but the blood is pale, boost the qi and stop bleeding by adding:

Radix Astragali Membranacei (*Huang Qi*)
Radix Codonopsis Pilosulae (*Dang Shen*)
Rhizoma Atractylodis Macrocephalae (*Bai Zhu*)
Rhizoma Cimicifugae (*Sheng Ma*)
Gelatinum Corii Asini (*E Jiao*)

If there is a history of habitual miscarriage, warm the kidneys and consolidate the *chong* by adding:

Cortex Eucommiae Ulmoidis (*Du Zhong*)
Radix Dipsaci (*Xu Duan*)
Ramus Loranthi Seu Visci (*Sang Ji Sheng*)
Rhizoma Cibotii (*Gou Ji*)

Sun Ning-quan found that, based on research data, if phase I or the hypothermal phase is prolonged, this is due to either kidney yin vacuity or spleen vacuity. During phase II, the transition from hypo to hyperthermal states may be prolonged due to either kidney yin vacuity, kidney yang vacuity, spleen vacuity, or liver depression. This transitional period should only last less than 3 days. If it lasts more than 5 days, an ovulatory disorder is indicated. Maintenance of a normal hyperthermal phase premenstrually may be due to either kidney yang vacuity or liver depression. These statements help practitioners hone in on the key disease mechanisms during each phase of the menstrual cycle.

134

Of the 60 cases included in this study, the ages of the women went from 25-37 years old with an average age of 31. The duration of these women's infertility was from 1.5-8 years with an average of 3.5 years. Thirty-two cases had a simple luteal phase defect (LPD). Twenty-one cases had LPD plus fallopian tube complications. Three had antisperm antibodies. And 3 had husbands with abnormal sperm. Eleven patients had a history of spontaneous miscarriage. Four had premenstrual bleeding. And 3 had midcycle bleeding. Eighteen were diagnosed as suffering from kidney yin vacuity, 20 from kidney yang vacuity, 6 from spleen/kidney dual vacuity, and 15 from kidney vacuity, liver depression. Of the 32 cases of uncomplicated LPD, 18 conceived in 3-6 months for a success rate of 56%.

I have used this protocol and have found it quite good as long as modifications are made for individual presenting complications.

7. Yang Yang-sheng's Protocol for Luteal Phase Defect[7]

This protocol is also designed to treat luteal phase defect. Its treatment is timed with the menses. However, instead of administering medicinals throughout the cycle, only a single formula is given during 4 days of phase III. The formula used is a version of *Si Wu Tang*.

Rx: *Si Wu Tang*

Radix Angelicae Sinensis (*Dang Gui*)
Radix Albus Paeoniae Lactiflorae (*Bai Shao*)
Rhizoma Ligustici Wallichii (*Chuan Xiong*)
Radix Rubrus Paeoniae Lactiflorae (*Chi Shao*)

---

[7] Yang Yang-sheng, "Report on 40 Cases of Corpus Luteum Functional Deficiency Treated with *Si Wu Tang* as a Base Formula," *Zhong Yi Za Zhi (Journal of TCM)*, No. 10. 1986, p. 34-35

Radix Rehmanniae (*Sheng Di*)
prepared Radix Rehmanniae (*Shu Di*)

If there is kidney yang vacuity, add 1-2 of the following:

Semen Cuscutae (*Tu Si Zi*)
Fluoritum (*Zi Shi Ying*)
Rhizoma Curculiginis Orchoidis (*Xian Mao*)
Herba Epimedii (*Xian Ling Pi*)
Fructus Rubi (*Fu Pen Zi*)

If there is kidney yin vacuity, add 1-2 of the following:

Fructus Ligustri Lucidi (*Nu Zhen Zi*)
Fructus Schizandrae Chinensis (*Wu Wei Zi*)
Fructus Lycii Chinensis (*Gou Qi Zi*)
Radix Scrophulariae Ningpoensis (*Yuan Shen*)
Herba Ecliptae Prostratae (*Han Lian Cao*)
Tuber Ophiopogonis Japonicae (*Mai Dong*)

Administer 1 *ji* per day during the 18th to 22nd days. Do not administer during menstruation.

Of the 27 cases treated with this protocol, 19 conceived after an average of 45 *ji*. Thirteen conceived within 3 months, 3 within 4-6 months, and 3 after more than 7 months of taking this formula. The overall pregnancy rate was 70.4% with only a 7.5% rate of miscarriage. This rate of miscarriage is close to that in the general population. This rate is specifically mentioned since a luteal phase defect means insufficient progesterone production and insufficient progesterone is a main reason for miscarriage. No birth defects were recorded among the babies of the mothers in this study. This helps show that Chinese medicinals are not teratogenic.

8. Xu Shang-yang's Protocol for Hyperestrogenosis, PMS, & Infertility[8]

Xu Shang-yang studied 140 cases of female infertility. Of these, 84 or 60% displayed signs and symptoms of liver depression, qi stagnation. These included premenstrual breast distention and pain, flank and lower abdominal distention and pain, chest oppression, frequent sighing, and a wiry pulse. Of these 84, 46 showed a luteal phase defect based on their BBT. The following therapeutic principles and formula were used to treat these women.

Therapeutic principles: Course the liver and resolve depression, supplement the kidneys and nourish the liver

Rx:

Radix Bupleuri (*Chai Hu*)
Fructus Meliae Toosendanis (*Chuan Lian Zi*)
prepared Radix Rehmanniae (*Di Huang*)
Fructus Rubi (*Fu Pen Zi*)
Tuber Curcumae (*Yu Jin*)
Fructus Citri Seu Ponciri (*Zhi Ke*)
Radix Morindae Officinalis (*Ba Ji Tian*)
Semen Cuscutae (*Tu Si Zi*)
Semen Citri Reticulatae (*Ju He*)
Radix Angelicae Sinensis (*Dang Gui*)
Fructus Lycii Chinensis (*Gou Qi Zi*)
Rhizoma Cyperi Rotundi (*Xiang Fu*)
Radix Albus Paeoniae Lactiflorae (*Bai Shao*)

---

[8] Xu Shang-yang, "A Study of the Relationship in Female Infertility Between Chinese Medical Differentiations and Basal Body Temperature and Endometrial Biopsy," *Shang Hai Zhong Yi Ya Za Zhi (Shanghai Journal of TCM)*, 1985, p. 22-23

Fructus Corni Officinalis (*Shan Zhu Yu*)

Tang does not report on the timing or number of *ji* administered per cycle nor the overall success rates. However, following this treatment for liver qi, serum estrogen levels decreased and these women's PMS symptoms were alleviated.

9. Pang Bao-zhen and Zhao Huan-yun's Protocol for Anovulation[9]

This protocol, published in 1992, describes the treatment of 149 women suffering from anovulatory infertility. Like many modern TCM infertility protocols, it assumes that kidney vacuity plays a role in most endocrine dyscrasias resulting in infertility. However, it is interesting because it compares a formula for simply supplementing the kidneys against one which supplements the kidneys and courses the liver.

In this study, 77 of the women were treated by supplementing the kidneys and coursing the liver. Of these, the duration of their complaint ranged from 2-19 years with most having suffered from 3-4 years. There were 26 cases of polycystic ovarian syndrome, 6 cases of anovulation with functional uterine bleeding, 16 cases of amenorrhea, 17 cases with anovulation and menstruation, and 12 cases of corpus luteum insufficiency.

Another 72 women were treated by supplementing the kidneys alone. Of these, the duration of their complaint ranged from 2-20 years with most having suffered between 3-4 years similar to the first group.

---

[9] Pang Bao-zhen & Zhao Huan-yun, "*Bu Shen Shu Gan He Bu Shen Zhi Liao Wu Pai Luan Xing Bu Yun 149 Li* (The Treatment of 149 Cases of Anovulatory Infertility by Supplementing the Kidneys and Coursing the Liver and by [Just Simply] Supplementing the Kidneys)", *Zhe Jiang Zhong Yi Za Zhi (Zhejiang Journal of TCM)*, No. 12, 1992, p. 539

Amongst these patients, 25 were diagnosed with polycystic ovarian syndrome, 5 with anovulation and functional uterine bleeding, 14 with amenorrhea, 18 with anovulation and menstruation, and 10 with corpus luteum insufficiency.

Rx: *Bu Shen Fang* (Kidney Supplementing Formula)

Fluoritum (*Zi Shi Ying*)
Fructus Zanthoxyli Bungeani (*Chuan Jiao*)
Radix Morindae Officinalis (*Ba Ji Tian*)
Fructus Lycii Chinensis (*Gou Qi Zi*)
Semen Cuscutae (*Tu Si Zi*)
Radix Dipsaci (*Chuan Duan*)
Herba Cistanchis (*Rou Cong Rong*)
prepared Radix Rehmanniae (*Shu Di*)

Bu Shen Shu Gan Fang (Kidney Supplementing, Liver Coursing Formula)

Same as above plus:

Radix Bupleuri (*Chai Hu*)
Rhizoma Cyperi Rotundi (*Xiang Fu*)
Fructus Citri Seu Ponciri (*Zhi Ke*)
Caulis Polygoni Multiflori (*Ye Jiao Teng*)

Beginning 5 days after the onset of menstruation, 6-10 *ji* or packets were administered, 1 per day. For those without a menstrual cycle, 3 *ji* were administered followed by 3 days halt. Another 3 *ji* were again followed by another 3 days halt, etc. The minimum duration of treatment was one month, the maximum was 6 months, and the average was 3 months.

Of the group receiving kidney supplementation alone, 40 experienced either complete cure or obvious improvement for a 55.56% amelioration rate. Within this group, amongst the 25 women with polycystic ovarian syndrome, 6 were cured, 8 experienced pronounced improvement, 6 experienced slight improvement, and 5 experienced no improvement. Of the 5 with anovulation and functional uterine bleeding, 1 experienced complete cure, 2 experienced pronounced improvement, and 2 experienced no improvement. Of the 14 with amenorrhea, 1 experienced complete cure, 2 pronounced improvement, 2 some improvement, and 9 no improvement. Of the 18 with anovulation and menstruation, 4 experienced complete cure, 6 pronounced improvement, and 8 no improvement. And of the 10 with corpus luteum insufficiency, 3 experienced complete cure and 7 pronounced improvement.

In the kidney supplementing and liver coursing group, of the 26 with polycystic ovarian syndrome, 8 experienced complete cure, 12 pronounced improvement, 3 some improvement, and 3 no improvement. Of the 6 with anovulation and functional uterine bleeding, 1 experienced complete cure, 2 pronounced improvement, and 3 no improvement. Of the 16 with amenorrhea, 2 experienced complete cure, 4 pronounced improvement, 3 some improvement, and 7 no improvement. Of the 17 with anovulation and menstruation, 7 experienced complete cure, 8 pronounced improvement, and 2 no improvement. And of the 12 with corpus luteum insufficiency, 5 experienced complete cure and another 7 pronounced improvement.

These results suggest that this protocol is not very effective for treating amenorrhea. Although the liver coursing ingredients, in this case, help, the results are still not very good. Nor does the kidney supplementing protocol seem very effective for treating anovulation and menstruation. In that case, the liver coursing medicinals seem to make a big difference. In fact, the overall results of this comparative study suggest that supplementing the kidneys alone is not categorically sufficient for the treatment of female infertility. The simultaneous coursing of the liver and rectifying of the qi resulted in an additional almost 20% amelioration rate.

Not only does this study emphasize the importance of coursing the liver and rectifying the qi in the treatment of female infertility, it also implicitly emphasizes the importance of basing treatment on a TCM *bian zheng* diagnosis. The women in this study were randomized without taking into account their TCM pattern diagnosis. Although most women in this protocol were benefitted if only slightly, a significant number received no benefit at all. For me, this study highlights the importance of making a individual *bian zheng* diagnosis and administering treatment on the basis of such a diagnosis and not solely on some abstract concept that female infertility always includes an element of kidney vacuity.

10. Li Dan's Protocol for Luteal Phase Defect[10]

This protocol published in 1992 discusses the treatment of corpus luteum defect with infertility in 46 women by supplementing the kidneys and coursing depression. Among these women, 4 were between the ages of 22-24, 35 were between 25-30, and 7 were between 31-36. Thirty-nine suffered from primary infertility and the other 7 from secondary infertility. Thirty-three had not been able to conceive in 2 years of trying and 13 had not been able to conceive in 3 years or more.

Based on a TCM *bian zheng* diagnosis, 32 of these women were categorized as kidney yang vacuous. This represented 69.9% of the total number of cases; while 14 cases were categorized as kidney yin vacuous or 30.4%. These women all experienced hyperthermal phases of less than 12 days duration. The temperature during their hyperther-

---

[10] Li Dan, *"Bu Shen Shu Yu Fa Zhi Liao Huang Ti Bu Jian Bu Yun 46 Li* (The Treatment of 46 Cases of Corpus Luteum Defect Infertility with Kidney-supplementing, Liver-coursing Methods)," *He Nan Zhong Yi (Henan Traditional Chinese Medicine)*, Vol. 12, No. 6, Nov. 1992, p. 281-282

mal phase fluctuated in excess of 0.1°C to 0.3°C. And their transition phase lasted more than 3 days.

All 46 women were treated with the same formula based on the principles of supplementing the kidneys and coursing depression.

Rx: *Bu Shen Shu Yu Tang*

Cornu Degelatinum Cervi (*Lu Jiao Shuang*)
Radix Morindae Officinalis (*Ba Ji Tian*)
Herba Cistanchis (*Rou Cong Rong*)
Radix Dipsaci (*Chuan Duan*)
Semen Vaccariae Segetalis (*Wang Bu Liu Xing*)
Fructus Ligustri Lucidi (*Nu Zhen Zi*)
Fructus Lycii Chinensis (*Gou Qi Zi*)
Semen Pruni Persicae (*Tao Ren*)
Flos Carthami Tinctorii (*Hong Hua*)
stir-fried Radix Albus Paeoniae Lactiflorae (*Bai Shao*)
Radix Dioscoreae Oppositae (*Shan Yao*)
processed Fructus Citri Seu Ponciri (*Zhi Ke*)
Radix Bupleuri (*Chai Hu*)
Radix Glycyrrhizae (*Sheng Gan Cao*)

Additions & subtractions based on pattern discrimination: After the period, add Radix Rehmanniae (*Sheng Di*) and prepared Radix Rehmanniae (*Shu Di*). In the intermenstrual phase, add Placenta Hominis (*Zi He Che*). Before the period, add Herba Epimedii (*Xian Ling Pi*). For those categorized as kidney yang vacuous, add Fluoritum (*Zi Shi Ying*), Placenta Hominis (*Zi He Che*), Radix Cibotti (*Gou Ji*), and Fructus Rubi (*Fu Pen Zi*). For those categorized as kidney yin vacuous, add Herba Ecliptae Prostratae (*Han Lian Cao*), Tuber Ophiopogonis Japonicae (*Mai Dong*), and Flos Immaturus Sophorae Japonicae (*Huai Hua*).

Decoct the above medicinals in 200 ml of water. Administer 2 times per day. Begin taking 7 days after the onset of menstruation and cease administration during the menses itself. One whole menstrual cycle equals 1 course of treatment.

Of the 46 women treated according to this protocol, 6 conceived within 1-3 courses of treatment. Without exception, all of these were categorized as kidney yang vacuous. Eighteen conceived in 4-6 courses. Eight conceived in 7-9 courses. And 2 conceived after 10-12 courses. Thus the conception rate was 73.9%. Of the 12 women who did not conceive, the BBT of 8 of these was somewhat improved. Four women experienced no improvement. Thus the total amelioration rate was 91.3%.

The author of this protocol states that corpus luteum defect is one of the most common causes of female infertility. According to Western medical theory, this is related to the thalamus/pituitary hypophysis/ovarian axis. It is this axis which explains in Western medical terminology how mental/emotional factors (the thalamus or cerebral cortex) affects the ovaries via the pituitary hypophysis. According to TCM theory, the change from preovulation to postovulation is described as the transformation of yin into yang. However, if kidney vacuity fails to warm and liver depression fails to course, the transformation of yin into yang may be slow or retarded. Thus yang qi does not come up in time. This results in a defect in the corpus luteum or what is more commonly known in English as a luteal phase defect.

The last two protocols above are important because they recognize and take into account the fact that liver depression commonly plays a part in most women's infertility due to endocrine dyscrasia. Due to stress, liver depression is a common complication in the very population of Western women who have deferred pregnancy until their late 30s and early 40s. In my experience, it is this very segment of the population that most commonly seeks help from Traditional Chinese Medicine for the treatment of their infertility.

11. Mao Qiu-zhi's Protocols for Luteal Phase Defect[11]

The corpus luteum is the yellow body left on the ovary after the ripened egg has been expressed. This site secretes progesterone which continues preparing the endometrium for implantation and forestalls menstruation. If there is a luteal defect, progesterone levels fall too low and typically the endometrium is shed too early. However, in some cases, it is the relative levels of progesterone and estrogen which are out of balance. In this case, it is hyperestrogenosis which is most pronounced and this can result in not only a host of premenstrual signs and symptoms but a delayed period as well.

In terms of female infertility, if there is a luteal phase defect with progesterone deficiency, even if there is a fertilized zygote, it cannot successfully implant and the endometrium is shed. This may be experienced as simply an early period. Or, if the egg has succeeded in implanting and pregnancy is confirmed, it may result in a miscarriage.

According to Hu Xi-ming in his preface to Mao Qiu-zhi's protocols for the treatment of luteal phase defect, the main TCM disease causes of this condition are insufficiency of kidney yin, deficiency and decline of kidney yang, and liver channel depressive heat. If there is kidney yin insufficiency, this may lead to early periods but with the amount of the menses not excessive. Its color is fresh red. Or menstruation may be prolonged with dribbling and dripping which will not stop. If kidney yang is vacuous and decrepit, this may lead to late periods which are sparse and scant and to infertility. Liver

---

[11]   Hu Xi-ming, *Zhong Guo Zhong Yi Mi Fang Da Quan (A Collaboration of Chinese TCM Secret Formulas)*, Literary Masterpieces Publication Co., Shanghai, 1992, p. 166-169

144

channel depressive heat leads to early, late, or periods occurring at no fixed schedule. Their amount is sometimes excessive and sometimes scant and they may continue on without being completely used up.

The treatment of this disease is to enrich and supplement kidney yin, stop the bleeding and regulate the menses for kidney yin vacuity. For kidney yang vacuity and decline, it is appropriate to treat the kidneys and strengthen yang, regulate and rectify the *chong* and *ren*. For liver channel depressive heat, one should course the liver, clear heat, and regulate and regulate the menses.

Rx: *Cu Huang Ti Tang*

prepared Radix Rehmanniae (*Shu Di*)
Plastrum Testudinis (*Gui Ban*)
Rhizoma Atractylodis Macrocephalae (*Bai Zhu*)
Radix Dipsaci (*Xu Duan*)
Herba Cistanchis (*Rou Cong Rong*)
stir-fried Flos Immaturus Sophorae Japonicae (*Huai Hua*)
Radix Angelicae Sinensis (*Dang Gui*)

Additions & subtractions based on pattern discrimination: For kidney yin vacuity, add Fructus Ligustri Lucidi (*Nu Zhen Zi*), and Herba Ecliptae Prostratae (*Han Lian Cao*). For kidney yang vacuity, add Radix Astragali Membranacei (*Huang Qi*), and Radix Morindae Officinalis (*Ba Ji Tian*).

This formula supplements the liver and kidneys, nourishes the *chong* and *ren*, and strengthens the corpus luteum. It is used to treat corpus luteal defect leading to loss of regulation and harmony of menstruation and infertility. It is given from the 17th to 25th days of the cycle.

Pai Luan Tang

Radix Bupleuri (*Chai Hu*)

Radix Rubrus Paeoniae Lactiflorae (*Chi Shao*)
Radix Albus Paeoniae Lactiflorae (*Bai Shao*)
Herba Lycopi Lucidi (*Ze Lan*)
(*Kun Cao*) (坤草)
Radix Angelicae Anomalae (*Liu Ji Nu*)
Caulis Millettiae Seu Spatholobi (*Ji Xue Teng*)
Radix Polygoni Multiflori (*Shou Wu*)
Pollen Typhae (*Sheng Pu Huang*)
Radix Dipsaci (*Chua Duan*)
Radix Achyranthis Bidentatae (*Niu Xi*)
Fructus Ligustri Lucidi (*Nu Zhen Zi*)
Herba Ecliptae Prostratae (*Han Lian Cao*)
Gelatinum Corii Asini (*E Jiao*)

This formula supplements the kidneys and regulates the liver, nourishes and quickens the blood. It treats corpus luteal defect with sparse, scanty menstruation and amenorrhea due to lack of ovulation. One hundred women were treated with this formula. Of those, 31 suffered from luteal phase defect, 28 from scanty, sparse menstruation, 28 from secondary amenorrhea, and 3 from primary amenorrhea. Of these 100 women, 25 conceived, 46 had their condition improve, and 29 experienced no result.

Bu Shen Si Wu Tang

Radix Angelicae Sinensis (*Dang Gui*)
Rhizoma Ligustici Wallichii (*Chuan Xiong*)
Radix Rubrus Paeoniae Lactiflorae (*Chi Shao*)
Radix Albus Paeoniae Lactiflorae (*Bai Shao*)
prepared Radix Rehmanniae (*Shu Di*)
Radix Rehmanniae (*Sheng Di*)

Additions & subtractions based on pattern discrimination: For kidney yang vacuity, add Fluoritum (*Zi Shi Ying*), Rhizoma Curculiginis Orchoidis (*Xian Mao*), Herba Epimedii (*Xian Ling Pi*), Semen

Cuscutae (*Tu Si Zi*), and Fructus Rubi (*Fu Pen Zi*). For kidney yin vacuity, add Fructus Ligustri Lucidi (*Nu Zhen Zi*), Herba Ecliptae Prostratae (*Han Lian Cao*), Fructus Lycii Chinensis (*Gou Qi Zi*), Fructus Schizandrae Chinensis (*Wu Wei Zi*), Radix Scrophulariae Ningpoensis (*Yuan Shen*), and Tuber Ophiopogonis Japonicae (*Mai Dong*).

This formula nourishes and quickens the blood, enriches and supplements kidney yin, warms and supplements kidney yang. It treats luteal phase defect and miscarriage due to progesterone deficiency.

When taking this formula, one menstrual cycle equals one course of treatment. Of 27 women treated with this formula, 19 conceived. Thirteen of these conceived after 3 months of treatment, 3 more after 4-6 months of treatment, and another 3 after 7 whole months of treatment. This equals a total conception rate of 70.4% with this formula.

Jian Quan Huang Ti Tang

Radix Dipsaci (*Xu Duan*)
Ramus Loranthi Seu Visci (*Sang Ji Sheng*)
Semen Cuscutae (*Tu Si Zi*)
Herba Leonuri Heterophylli (*Yi Mu Cao*)
Radix Rubrus Paeoniae Lactiflorae (*Chi Shao*)
Radix Albus Paeoniae Lactiflorae (*Bai Shao*)
Radix Scutellariae Baicalensis (*Huang Qin*)
Fasciculus Vascularis Luffae (*Si Gua Luo*)
processed Rhizoma Cyperi Rotundi (*Xiang Fu*)

This formula supplements the kidneys, quickens the blood, and opens the connecting vessels. It treats luteal phase defect, delayed ovulation, and lack of ovulation resulting in loss of regulation of the menses. Of 22 women treated with this formula, 66% conceived.

Personally, I do not think any of these three protocols take into sufficient account spleen qi vacuity's role in luteal phase defect infertility. Although, under the modifications for *Cu Huang Ti Tang*, Radix Astragali Membranacei (*Huang Qi*) is recommended for kidney yang vacuity, I think this issue needs to be addressed in more depth. In my experience, there is frequently concomitant yin and yang vacuity complicated by spleen qi vacuity resulting in a shortened hyperthermal phase, early periods, and inability to conceive. In such cases simply nourishing yin and clearing heat does not result in lengthened cycles. In my experience, this approach alone may shorten the cycle even more. Therefore, the right result is often brought about by adding qi supplements and boosters, such as Radix Astragali Membranacei, Radix Panacis Ginseng (*Ren Shen*), Radix Bupleuri (*Chai Hu*), and Rhizoma Cimicifugae (*Sheng Ma*).

12. Cao Ling-xian's Protocols for Midcycle Bleeding[12]

Although uterine bleeding during ovulation is not *per se* a cause of infertility, it is a symptom of hormonal dyscrasia. It is not uncommon to encounter women suffering from infertility who complain of persistent midcycle bleeding. By rectifying this bleeding, one can help rebalance the endocrine system and thus promote conception. Therefore, some knowledge about the mechanisms behind and treatment of midcycle bleeding is necessary for those who would treat female infertility.

Hu Xi-ming, in his preface to these three protocols, says that uterine bleeding during ovulation is traditionally categorized as early period or red and white abnormal vaginal discharge in TCM. This condition is mostly due to loss of balance between viscera and bowel function and the *chong* and *ren*. After the period, yin and blood are empty. The body attempts to replenish these as its first priority during the

---

[12] *Ibid.*, p. 170-172

148

proliferative phase. However, by midcycle, this growth of yin may give rise to a sudden spurt in the transformation of yang. At this point, yang may become relatively excessive with kidney yin and yang coming out of balance. If kidney yin is insufficient to restrain yang the *chong* and *ren* may be damaged and the connecting vessels injured. This may be complicated by depressive heat and/or damp heat hidden within the *chong* and *ren*. In that case, the blood vessels may be injured and blood may exit.

Treatment of this condition is mainly aimed at supplementing the kidneys and boosting yin at the same time as clearing vacuity fire within the kidneys. If there is damp heat, it is appropriate to supplement and boost the liver and kidneys, clear heat and eliminate dampness, dispel stasis and stop bleeding.

Rx: *Yang Shi Tiao Chong Tang*

Phase I

prepared Radix Rehmanniae (*Shu Di*)
Radix Dioscoreae Oppositae (*Shan Yao*)
Fructus Corni Officinalis (*Shan Zhu Rou*)
Semen Cuscutae (*Tu Si Zi*)
Herba Epimedii (*Xian Ling Pi*)
Radix Dipsaci (*Xu Duan*)
carbonized Radix Rehmanniae (*Sheng Di*)
stir-fried Radix Astragali Membranacei (*Huang Qi*)

Phase II

stir-fried Cortex Radicis Moutan (*Dan Pi*)
carbonized Radix Rehmanniae (*Sheng Di*)
Radix Bupleuri (*Chai Hu*)
Tuber Curcumae (*Yu Jin*)
Radix Albus Paeoniae Lactiflorae (*Bai Shao*)

Rhizoma Imperatae Cyclindricae (*Bai Mao Geng*)

Additions & subtractions based on pattern discrimination: For kidney vacuity, add Fructus Corni Officinalis (*Shan Zhu Rou*) and Herba Ecliptae Prostratae (*Mo Han Lian*). For spleen vacuity, add Radix Astragali Membranacei (*Huang Qi*), Sclerotium Poriae Cocoris (*Fu Ling*), and Pericarpium Citri Reticulatae (*Chen Pi*).

This formula supplements the kidneys and regulates the *chong*, courses the liver and cools the blood. It treats uterine bleeding during ovulation. The first formula should be taken during the proliferative phase after menstruation. The second formula should be taken during ovulation if bleeding occurs. Of 12 women treated with this formula, 11 were cured and the other was ameliorated.

Bu Shen Qing Re Fang

Radix Rehmanniae (*Sheng Di*)
Fructus Lycii Chinensis (*Qi Zi*)
Radix Dioscoreae Oppositae (*Shan Yao*)
Radix Albus Paeoniae Lactiflorae (*Bai Shao*)
Radix Glycyrrhizae (*Gan Cao*)
Herba Ecliptae Prostratae (*Mo Han Lian*)
Cortex Phellodendri (*Huang Bai*)
Radix Sophorae Flavescentis (*Ku Shen*)
Semen Nelumbinis Nuciferae (*Shi Lian Zi*)
Os Sepiae Seu Sepiellae (*Wu Zei Gu*)
Radix Rubiae Cordifoliae (*Qian Cao*)
carbonized Radix Angelicae Sinensis (*Dang Gui*)
Flos Celosiae Cristatae (*Ji Guan Hua*)

This formula supplements and boosts kidney yin, clears heat and eliminates dampness. It treats uterine bleeding during ovulation.

Wen Jing San Leng Qian

Flos Carthami Tinctorii (*Hong Hua*)
Radix Salviae Miltiorrhizae (*Dan Shen*)
Rhizoma Sparganii (*San Leng*)
Rhizoma Curcumae Zedoariae (*E Zhu*)
Ramulus Cinnamomi (*Gui Zhi*)
Radix Polygoni Multiflori (*Shou Wu*)
Radix Achyranthis Bidentatae (*Niu Xi*)
Fructus Crataegi (*Shan Zha*)
Feces Trogopterori Seu Pteromi (*Wu Ling Zhi*)
Fructus Evodiae Rutecarpae (*Wu Yu*)
Pulvis Corticis Cinnamomi (*Rou Gui Fen*)
Radix Saussureae Seu Vladimiriae (*Guang Mu Xiang*)

Administer during phase I, the postmenstruum.

Angelicae Sinensis (*Dang Gui*)
Rhizoma Cyperi Rotundi (*Xiang Fu*)
Gelatinum Corii Asini (*E Jiao*)
Radix Rubrus Paeoniae Lactiflorae (*Chi Shao*)
Radix Albus Paeoniae Lactiflorae (*Bai Shao*)
Concha Ostreae (*Mu Li*)
Os Sepiae Seu Sepiellae (*Wu Zei Gu*)
carbonized Cacumen Biotae Orientalis (*Ce Bai*)
carbonized Nodus Nelumbinis Nuciferae (*Ou Jie*)
Fructus Pruni Mume (*Wu Mei*)
mix-fried Radix Et Rhizoma Rhei (*Jun*)

Administer during phase II, ovulation.

When normalcy is achieved, in order to regulate and supplement the qi and blood, use:

Radix Rehmanniae (*Sheng Di*)
Herba Epimedii (*Xian Ling Pi*)

Fructus Psoraleae Corylifoliae (*Bu Gu Zhi*)
Radix Angelicae Sinensis (*Dang Gui*)
Rhizoma Cyperi Rotundi (*Xiang Fu*)
Fructus Ligustri Lucidi (*Nu Zhen*)
Herba Ecliptae Prostratae (*Han Lian*)
Radix Salviae Miltiorrhizae (*Dan Shen*)
Rhizoma Corydalis Yanhusuo (*Yan Hu*)
Pericarpium Citri Reticulatae (*Chen Pi*)

This protocol warms the kidneys and courses the liver, regulates and supplements yin and yang. It treats uterine bleeding during ovulation. One case of midcycle bleeding was treated with the above which had persisted for 3 years and had not responded to other treatments. After taking the above, the woman was cured.

13. Yu Shi's Protocol for Premature Ovarian Failure[13]

Hypothyroidism is a common cause of female infertility, and the most common cause of primary hypothyroidism is chronic inflammation of the thyroid with lymphocytic infiltration of the gland due to autoimmune factors. We will discuss further autoimmune issues as they relate to female infertility under candidiasis. However, Yu Shi gives a protocol for premature ovarian failure (*luan chao zao shuai*). This refers to menopause below the age of 40. Women with this condition present with signs and symptoms of estrogen deficiency and commonly have elevated circulating levels of gonadotropins, especially follicle stimulating hormone (FSH), and low levels of estradiol. Many cases of premature ovarian failure occur in association with other autoimmune disorders, such as thyroiditis, hypoparathyroidism, hypoadrenalism, diabetes mellitus, rheumatoid arthritis, myasthenia gravis, and pernicious anemia.

---

[13]   *Ibid.*, p. 195-197

In order to enrich yin and descend fire, supplement the kidneys and quicken the blood, Yu suggests the following formula.

Rx: *Luan Chao Zao Shuai Fang*

Rhizoma Anemarrhenae (*Zhi Mu*)
Cortex Phellodendri (*Huang Bai*)
Radix Rehmanniae (*Sheng Di*)
Plastrum Testudinis (*Gui Ban*)
Carapax Amydae (*Bei Jia*)
Fructus Ligustri Lucidi (*Nu Zhen Zi*)
Herba Epimedii (*Xian Ling Pi*)
Fructus Psoraleae Corylifoliae (*Bu Gu Zhi*)
Radix Rubrus Paeoniae Lactiflorae (*Chi Shao*)
Semen Pruni Persicae (*Tao Ren*)
Radix Angelicae Sinensis (*Dang Gui*)

Additions & subtractions based on pattern discrimination: If there is lack of strength, add Radix Pseudostellariae (*Tai Zi Shen*). If there are heart palpitations and one is easily angered, add Cortex Radicis Moutan (*Dan Pi*) and stir-fried Fructus Gardeniae Jasminoidis (*Shan Zhi*).

Six cases of premature ovarian failure were treated with this formula. These women's FSH levels dropped to normal after several months of therapy in all cases. Two women subsequently conceived.

6

Fallopian Tube Blockage

Fallopian tube blockage is frequently a sequela of salpingitis or inflammation of the fallopian tubes. Salpingitis may be either acute or chronic and is most often encountered in women under 25 years of age who are sexually active. This suggests that this inflammation is primarily due to infection transmitted through sexual intercourse. *Neisseria gonorrhea* is the responsible organism in 40-60% of acute nonpuerperal pelvic inflammatory disease. Other pathological organisms involved include *Chlamydia trachomatis*, gram-negative bacilli, gram-positive cocci, mycoplasmas, and viruses. When salpingitis follows pregnancy or abortion, anaerobic streptococci or staphylococci are usually involved. Tubal infection produces a profuse exudate and leads to agglutination of the mucosal folds, adhesions, and tubal occlusion. An obstructed tube may be distended with fluid. This is referred to as hydrosalpinx.

1. Dai Ting-tao's Protocol[1]

This protocol is designed to treat infertility due to blocked fallopian tubes. It uses four primary groups of medicinals, all of which assume that blocked fallopian tubes are due to stasis and stagnation. The groups of medicinals are as follows:

---

[1] Dai Ting-tao, "Clinical Experiences in the Cure of 23 Cases of Fallopian Tube Blockage Infertility," *Shang Hai Yi Yao Za Zhi (Shanghai Journal of TCM)*, No. 2, 1992, p. 9-10

155

1. To quicken the blood and rectify the qi:

Radix Angelicae Sinensis (*Dang Gui*)
Rhizoma Ligustici Wallichii (*Chuan Xiong*)
Radix Rubrus Paeoniae Lactiflorae (*Chi Shao*)
Radix Salviae Miltiorrhizae (*Dan Shen*)
Fructus Liquidambaris Taiwaniae (*Lu Lu Tong*)
Rhizoma Cyperi Rotundi (*Xiang Fu*)
Fructus Meliae Toosendanis (*Chuan Lian Zi*)
Radix Linderae Strychnifoliae (*Wu Yao*), etc.

2. To open the channels and transform stasis:

Flos Rosae Chinensis (*Yue Ji Hua*)
Herba Leonuri Heterophylli (*Yi Mu Cao*)
Semen Pruni Persicae (*Tao Ren*)
Flos Carthami Tinctorii (*Hong Hua*)
Rhizoma Sparganii (*San Leng*)
Rhizoma Curcumae Zedoariae (*E Zhu*)
Radix Et Rhizoma Rhei (*Da Huang*), etc.

3. To search, pick out, and open the *luo*:

Squama Manitis (*Chuan Shan Jia*)
Spina Gleditschiae (*Jiao Ci*)
Eupolyphagae Seu Opisthoplatiae (*Di Bie Chong*)
Scolopendrae Subspinipis (*Wu Gong*), etc.

4. To soften the hard and scatter nodulation:

Herba Sargassi (*Hai Zao*)
Thallus Algae (*Kun Bu*)
Concha Ostreae (*Sheng Mu Li*)
Rhizoma Dioscoreae Bulbiferae (*Huang Yao Zi*), etc.

Because the disease mechanisms assumed operative in this condition are all species of repletion, attacking therapies are predominant. In clinical practice the common signs and symptoms accompanying this condition are premenstrual breast distention and pain, lower abdominal distention and pain with the onset of the period, lumbosacral soreness and pain, a dark tongue with ecchymotic spots or patches, etc. Dai Ting-tao gives the following modifications for additions to the above medicinals.

Additions & subtractions based on pattern discrimination: If qi and blood are vacuous and weak, add Radix Codonopsis Pilosulae (*Dang Shen*), Radix Astragali Membranacei (*Huang Qi*), prepared Radix Rehmanniae (*Shu Di*), Fructus Lycii Chinensis (*Gou Qi*), etc. If liver and kidneys are insufficient, add Fructus Corni Officinalis (*Shan Zhu Yu*), Plastrum Testudinis (*Gui Ban*), Semen Cuscutae (*Tu Si Zi*), Fructus Rubi (*Fu Pen Zi*), Herba Epimedii (*Xian Ling Pi*), Radix Morindae Officinalis (*Ba Ji Tian*), etc. If the spleen and stomach are vacuous and weak, add Rhizoma Atractylodis Macrocephalae (*Bai Zhu*), Radix Dioscoreae Oppositae (*Shan Yao*), Pericarpium Citri Reticulatae (*Chen Pi*), Fructus Amomi (*Sha Ren*), etc. If the liver is depressed and qi is stagnant, add Radix Bupleuri (*Chai Hu*), Tuber Curcumae (*Yu Jin*), Fructus Citri Seu Ponciri (*Zhi Ke*), Pericarpium Viridis Citri Reticulatae (*Qing Pi*), etc. If there is phlegm dampness, add Rhizoma Pinelliae Ternatae (*Ban Xia*), Sclerotium Poriae Cocoris (*Fu Ling*), Rhizoma Arisaematis (*Nan Xing*), Semen Plantaginis (*Che Qian Zi*), etc.

These basic recommendations are then coordinated with the phases of the menstrual cycle.

Phase I & II

Therapeutic principles: Quicken the blood and transform stasis, search, pick out, and open the *luo*, soften the hard and scatter nodulation,

157

and, as appropriate, regulate and supplement yin and yang, qi and blood

Rx: If there is longstanding blockage and inflammation, especially use

Squama Manitis (*Chuan Shan Jia*)
Eupolyphagae Seu Opisthoplatiae (*Tu Bie Chong*)
Scolopendra Subspinipes (*Wu Gong*)
Fructus Liquidambaris Taiwaniae (*Lu Lu Tong*)
Spina Gleditschiae (*Jiao Ci*), etc.

Quickening the blood and transforming stasis medicinals are able to disperse inflammation and disperse swelling.

Phase III

Therapeutic principles: Either supplement the kidneys and nourish the liver, boost the qi and nourish the blood, or course the liver and rectify the qi as necessary

Phase IV

Therapeutic principles: Quicken the blood and move the qi

Rx: Primarily use medicinals which quicken the blood and move the qi plus

Flos Rosae Chinensis (*Yue Ji Hua*) or
Radix Et Rhizoma Rhei (*Da Huang*)
Semen Pruni Persicae (*Tao Ren*)
Flos Carthami Tinctorii (*Hong Hua*)
Herba Leonuri Heterophylli (*Yi Mu Cao*)
Rhizoma Sparganii (*San Leng*)
Rhizoma Curcumae Zedoariae (*E Zhu*), etc.

If there is chronic salpingitis, use 20-30g of Flos Rosae Chinensis. The *Ben Cao Gang Mu (The Detailed OUtline of the Materia Medica)* says, "(Its) qi and flavor are sweet and warm, without toxicity; (it) primarily treats by quickening the blood, disperses swelling, and is sufficient for toxins." Administer such medicinals from days 1-3, 1 *ji* per day.

Although this protocol does not give actual formulas, it is, nonetheless, interesting and useful. It deals with a nonhumoral cause of infertility. Yet it still uses the phases of the menses to guide the treatment plan with the same TCM rationale during each phase as in the above protocols. This helps underscore the importance of understanding the key issues, both normal and pathological, during each phase of the cycle. Thus side effects due to erroneous treatment given at the wrong time are guarded against and maximum efficacy is achieved therapeutically by working with the body's own inherent processes and rhythms.

Dai reports that 23 infertile women with fallopian tube blockage were treated with this protocol. Of these, both tubes were blocked in 18 cases and only one tube was blocked in 5 cases. Seven cases were under 30 years of age. Twelve cases were between 30-34, and 4 cases were over 35. The minimum time any patient had been infertile was 2 years and the maximum was 6 years. It is stated that the minimum cure time was 2 months and the maximum was more than 1 year.

2. Cui Wen-qing's Protocol[2]

This protocol published in 1992 is for infertility due to fallopian tube blockage and uses a three stage treatment coordinated with the menstrual cycle.

---

[2] Cui Wen-qing, "The Treatment of 100 Cases of Fallopian Tube Blockage and Infertility," *Shang Hai Zhong Yi Yao Za Zhi (Shanghai Journal of TCM)*, No. 3, 1992, p. 19-20

From days 1-10 of the menstrual cycle, the following formula is administered:

Caulis Sargentodoxae (*Hong Teng*)
Flos Lonicerae Japonicae (*Yin Hua*)
Semen Pruni Persicae (*Tao Ren*)
Radix Angelicae Sinensis (*Dang Gui*)
Rhizoma Ligustici Wallichii (*Chuan Xiong*)
Rhizoma Cyperi Rotundi (*Xiang Fu*)
Tuber Ophiopogonis Japonicae (*Mai Dong*)
Semen Coicis Lachryma-jobi (*Sheng Mi Ren*)
Pulvis Radicis Pseudoginseng (*San Qi Fen*), swallowed separately

From days 11-20, administer the following formula:

Radix Angelicae Sinensis (*Dang Gui*)
Radix Rubrus Paeoniae Lactiflorae (*Chi Shao*)
Radix Salviae Miltiorrhizae (*Dan Shen*)
Carapax Praeparatus Amydae (*Zhi Jia Pian*)
Radix Scrophulariae Ningpoensis (*Xuan Shen*)
Caulis Sargentodoxae (*Hong Teng*)
Herba Cum Radice Taraxaci Mongolici (*Pu Gong Ying*)
Hirudo Seu Whitmaniae (*Shui Zhi*)
Rhizoma Curcumae Zedoariae (*E Zhu*)
Feces Trogopterori Seu Pteromi (*Wu Ling Zhi*)
Pulvis Radicis Pseudoginseng (*San Qi Fen*), swallowed separately

From days 21-30, administer the following formula:

Flos Lonicerae Japonicae (*Yin Hua*)
Herba Patriniae Heterophyllae (*Bai Jiang Cao*)
Caulis Millettiae Seu Spatholobi (*Ji Xue Teng*)
Rhizoma Cyperi Rotundi (*Xiang Fu*)
Fructus Rosae Laevigatae (*Jin Ying Zi*)
Folium Daqingye (*Da Qing Ye*)

160

Radix Rubiae Cordifoliae (*Qian Cao*)
Herba Leonuri Heterophylli (*Yi Mu Cao*)
Rhizoma Corydalis Yanhusuo (*Xuan Hu*)
Semen Zanthoxyli Bungeani (*Chuan Jiao Zi*)
Pulvis Radicis Pseudoginseng (*San Qi Fen*), swallowed separately

Three whole months equal one course of treatment and most women in the study utilizing this protocol received from one to two such courses. Fifty women were treated with these three formulas, all of whom suffered from fallopian tube blockage and infertility. They ranged in age from a low of 24 to a high of 39 years old. Of these, 33 suffered from primary infertility and 17 from secondary infertility. In other words, 33 had never conceived in their life, while 17 had conceived previously but had not been able to conceive again after 3 years of trying. Thirty-six women or 72% subsequently were cured, meaning that they conceived. Another 7 women or 14% received partial benefit. This means that their fallopian tubes were no longer blocked but they did not conceive. Four women or 8% had one of their tubes unblocked while the other remained blocked, and 3 women or 6% received no benefit at all.

This protocol is based on the principles of quickening the blood and transforming stasis, clearing heat and resolving toxins. This is based on the underlying assumption that fallopian tube blockage is often due to blood stasis mutually binding and wrestling with dampness and heat or even hot toxins. In my experience, this is an often encountered pattern in Western women.

I also find some elegant touches in this protocol. For instance, in the proliferative phase, Tuber Ophiopogonis Japonicae is added to clear heat from the heart and to nourish yin fluids. This is based on Li Dong-yuan's theory of yin fire. If damp heat smolders below, the heat will have a tendency to waft up along the *bao mai/chong mai* to collect in the heart where it wastes and injures yin fluids. Most cyclically phased protocols assume the necessity of supplementing yin after the period. However, this protocol nourishes heart and stomach yin as opposed to the more commonly supplemented kidney yin.

During what would correspond to the ovulatory phase, this protocol follows modern Chinese suit by emphasizing the quickening of the blood and transformation of stasis. However, it does also address the resolution of toxins due to exacerbation of heat at midcyle. In addition, it clears vacuity heat above with the addition of Carapax Amydae and Radix Scrophulariae Ningpoensis.

During the premenstruum, this protocol continues to clear heat and eliminate dampness and toxins, quicken the blood and transform stasis. Nonetheless, by adding Fructus Rosae Laevigatae, an astringent medicinal which supplements kidney qi, Semen Zanthoxyli Bungeani, a warming ingredient which warms the kidneys and aids yang, and Caulis Millettiae Seu Spatholobi, an ingredient which quickens the channels and relaxes the sinews but also treats wind damp obstruction, this formula simultaneously addresses the tendency for damp heat to coexist and even cause kidney yang vacuity.

When such yang vacuity is coexistent with damp heat in the lower burner, it does typically worsen before the period. Since damp heat often enters the blood level, women with damp heat and yang vacuity commonly experience early periods due to a combination of both heat causing the blood to run recklessly outside its pathways and the kidneys being insufficient to astringe the lower yin. I believe that such a tendency to early menstruation is the reason for the addition of Radix Rubiae Cordifoliae at this stage. This medicinal clears heat and stops bleeding while at the same time quickening the blood and transforming stasis.

This protocol addresses a fairly complicated scenario. The same mechanisms are often at work in many Western women's endometriosis and the infertility which that condition also causes.

3. Yue Xiu-zhen *et al.*'s Protocol[3]

This protocol published in 1992 involves the treatment of 100 cases of infertility due to fallopian tube blockage. It does not use a phased approach to treatment as the above protocols do. However, it is interesting because it compares treatment with orally administered Chinese medicinals alone with oral and anally administered Chinese herbs and with orally administered herbs and histosalpingogram.

Rx for oral administration:

Fructus Meliae Toosendanis (*Chuan Lian Zi*)
Fructus Citri Seu Ponciri (*Zhi Ke*)
Pericarpium Viridis Citri Reticulatae (*Qing Pi*)
Pericarpium Citri Reticulatae (*Chen Pi*)
Herba Pycnostelmae (*Xu Chang Qing*), etc.

One *ji* of the above was given in 1 dose per day. Treatment was suspended during the period itself. Herba Pycnostelmae is acrid and warm, removes wind and eliminates dampness, resolves toxins, and disperses swelling. It is indicated for hernial and uterine pain as well as for rheumatic complaints.

Rx for administration by enema:

Caulis Lonicerae (*Ren Dong Teng*)
Herba Verbenae Officinalis (*Ma Bian Cao*)
Spina Gleditschiae (*Jiao Ci*)
Radix Glycyrrhizae (*Sheng Gan Cao*)

---

[3] Yue Xin-zhen *et al.*, "Observation on the Effects of Treatment of 100 Cases of Fallopian Tube Blockage Infertility," *Shang Hai Zhong Yi Yao Za Zhi (Shanghai Journal of TCM)*, No. 3, 1992, p. 19-20

Use 1 *ji* of the above daily for 10 days beginning 3 days after the cessation of menstruation.

In the third group, salt water was injected into their uterus and up into their fallopian tubes during phases I and II, once per day for 10 days. Three months of this treatment was considered one course of therapy. Six of the 23 women who took the oral Chinese medicinals alone conceived after 6 months of therapy for a 20.69% success rate. Twenty-one out of the 38 women who took Chinese medicinals both orally and anally conceived for a 55.26% success rate, and 15 out of the 33 women who took Chinese medicinals orally and had injection therapy conceived for a success rate of 45.45%. These statistics suggest that for fallopian tube blockage, anal administration of medicinals with oral administration is more than twice as effective as oral administration alone. This logic might also be used in the treatment of endometriosis.

4. Shi Jie-yu's Protocol[4]

In this protocol researched from mid-1989 to mid-1990, fallopian tube blockage in 37 women complaining of infertility was treated by Chinese medicinal enemas. Of these 37 women, 32 had never conceived. The ages of 19 of these women ranged between 25-30 years. Sixteen were between 31-35, and there were two women 36 years old or older. Eighteen had not been able to conceive within three years of trying, fifteen in 3-4 years of trying, and four in 4-5 years of trying. Further, eight suffered from bilateral obstruction of their tubes, ten suffered from obstruction of their ampullae, three cases suffered from hydrosalpinx, and sixteen suffered from pelvic adhesions and endometritis. Twenty-three women had previously tried Chinese herbal medicine for 6 months to 1 year with no result and the

---

[4]   Shi Jie-yu, "Retention Enema with Chinese Herbal Medicine for 37 Cases of Infertility Caused by Obstruction of Fallopian Tube," *Shang Hai Zhong Yi Yao Za Zhi (Shanghai Journal of TCM)*, No. 12, 1992, p. 13

other fourteen had tried Western medicine without result for around 6 months.

This protocol used two different formulas administered as retention enemas.

Rx: *Hong Teng Yi Hao Fang*

Caulis Sargentodoxae (*Hong Teng*)
Herba Violae Yedoensis (*Di Ding Cao*)
Herba Patriniae Heterophyllae (*Bai Jiang Cao*)
Herba Cum Radice Taraxaci Mongolici (*Pu Gong Ying*)
Herba Commelinae (*Ya Zhi Cao*)
Flos Carthami Tinctorii (*Hong Hua*)
Rhizoma Corydalis Yanhusuo (*Yan Hu*)
Rhizoma Cyperi Rotundi (*Xiang Fu*)
Liu Xing Zi (留行子)
Caulis Et Folium Lonicerae (*Ren Dong Teng*)

The composition of this formula is based on the principles of clearing heat and resolving toxins, rectifying the qi and opening the connecting vessels.

Hong Teng Er Hao Fang

Caulis Sargentodoxae (*Hong Teng*)
Rhizoma Polygoni Cuspidati (*Hu Chang*)
Herba Patriniae Heterophyllae (*Bai Jiang Cao*)
Radix Angelicae Sinensis (*Dang Gui*)
Radix Salviae Miltiorrhizae (*Dan Shen*)
Fructus Liquidambaris Taiwaniae (*Lu Lu Tong*)
Eupolyphagae Seu Opisthoplatiae (*Tu Bie Chong*)
Rhizoma Sparganii (*San Leng*)
Rhizoma Curcumae Zedoariae (*E Zhu*)
Feces Trogopterori Seu Pteromi (*Wu Ling Zhi*)

Pollen Typhae (*Pu Huang*)
Spina Gleditschiae Sinensis (*Jiao Ci*)
Radix Astragali Membranacei (*Sheng Huang Qi*)

The composition of this formula is based on the principles of quickening the blood and transforming stasis, softening the hard and scattering nodulation.

Each of these formulas was modified according to the disease and pattern. The medicinals were decocted down to between 80-100 milliliters. The resulting decoction was administered once per day even during the menses. Three months of therapy was considered one course of treatment. During the first month, *Hong Teng Yi Hao Fang* was administered. During the second and third months, *Hong Teng Er Hao Fang* was used. Patients in this study received 1-2 courses of treatment.

Thirty-two of the 37 so treated eventually conceived for a conception rate of 86.48%. Of these, 24 conceived after one course of treatment and another 8 after a second course. Five women did not conceive after two complete courses of treatment even though examination showed that their tubes were open and free-flowing.

Shi Jie-yu comments that because these formulas clear heat and resolve toxins and quicken the blood and transform stasis, they cannot be taken orally for a long period of time because they would damage the stomach qi. However, by administering them as an enema, this side effect is avoided. In addition, the medicine is absorbed by tissue adjacent to the target site of the medicinals' action.

5. Bei Run-pu's Protocol[5]

This protocol for infertility due to blocked fallopian tubes is based on research conducted on 150 women. After 1 year of treatment, 122 women's tubes were no longer blocked and 105 or 70% had conceived. The treatment principles used to design the treatment protocol were to transform stasis and soften the hard, disperse mass and move stasis, soothe and ease the *bao luo*, and course and open the fallopian tubes. A root formula was created based on these principles which was then modified depending upon the patients' individual complicating patterns.

Rx:

Radix Angelicae Sinensis (*Dang Gui*)
Herba Sargassi (*Hai Zao*)
Radix Glycyrrhizae (*Gan Cao*)
Squama Manitis (*Chuan Shan Jia*)
Semen Vaccariae Segetalis (*Wang Bu Liu Xing*)
Fructus Liquidambaris Taiwaniae (*Lu Lu Tong*)
Concha Ostreae (*Mu Li*)
Radix Achyranthis Bidentatae (*Niu Xi*)
Radix Clematidis (*Wei Ling Xian*)
Caulis Solani Lyrati (*Bai Mao Teng*)
Flos Rosae Chinensis (*Yue Ji Hua*)

Additions & subtractions based on pattern discrimination: If there is cold stasis, delete the Caulis Solani Lyrati and add Ramulus Cinnamomi (*Gui Zhi*), Herba Cum Radice Asari Sieboldi (*Xi Xin*), Semen Trigonellae Foeni-graeci (*Hu Lu Ba*), and/or Fructus Evodiae

---

[5] Bei Run-pu, "A Report on the Treatment of 150 Cases of Fallopian Tube Blockage and Subsequent Infertility," *Zhong Yi Za Zhi (Journal of TCM)*, No. 3, 1992, p. 20-22

Rutecarpae (*Wu Zhu Yu*). If there is stasis heat, delete Radix Clematidis and add Cortex Radicis Moutan (*Dan Pi*), Radix Salviae Miltiorrhizae (*Dan Shen*), Caulis Sargentodoxae (*Hong Teng*), Radix Rubrus Paeoniae Lactiflorae (*Chi Shao*), and/or Herba Patriniae Heterophyllae (*Bai Jiang Cao*). If there is liver depression, also delete Radix Clematidis and add Radix Bupleuri (*Chai Hu*), Fructus Akebiae (*Ba Yue Zha*), and Cornu Degelatinum Cervi (*Lu Jiao Shuang*). If there is qi vacuity, delete Radix Achyranthis Bidentatae and Flos Rosae Chinensis and add Radix Codonopsis Pilosulae (*Dang Shen*), Radix Astragali Membranacei (*Huang Qi*), and Semen Litchi Chinensis (*Li Zhi He*).

One *ji* of this formula is administered in 2 equal doses per day commencing 3 days after the cessation of menstruation and stopping 3 days before the onset of the next period. During the period itself, it is recommended to take *Si Zhi Xiang Fu Wan*. If the amount of menstruation is excessive, also administer the patent medicine *Zhen Ling Dan*. If the amount of the menses is scant and there is abdominal pain, administer *Da Huang Zhe Chong Wan* along with *Si Zhi Xiang Fu Wan*. If the basal body temperature shows that the luteal phase is comparatively short and both phases do not display the standard pattern or curve, in order to promote ovulation and strengthen the corpus luteum, one can also add medicinals such as:

Fructus Lycii Chinensis (*Gou Qi Zi*)
Herba Cistanchis (*Rou Cong Rong*)
Herba Epimedii (*Xian Ling Pi*)
Rhizoma Curculiginis Orchoidis (*Xian Mao*)
Semen Cuscutae (*Tu Si Zi*)
prepared Radix Rehmanniae (*Shu Di*)
Herba Dendrobii (*Shi Hu Ye*)
Semen Allii Tuberosi (*Jiu Cai Zi*)
Fructus Ligustri Lucidi (*Nu Zhen Zi*)
Radix Glycyrrhizae (*Gan Cao*) etc.

These are to be added to the above root formula and likewise given from the third day after the cessation of the period up to three days before the onset of the next period.

Like the protocol above, this one also uses an enema. It is composed of:

Herba Tougucao (*Tou Gu Cao*)
Spina Gleditschiae (*Jiao Ci*)
processed Gummum Olibanni (*Ru Xiang*)
processed Myrrha (*Mo Yao*)
Rhizoma Smilacis Glabrae (*Tu Fu Ling*)
Radix Clematidis (*Wei Ling Xian*)
Rhizoma Sparganii (*San Leng*)
Radix Sophorae Flavescentis (*Ku Shen*)

These ingredients are decocted in 100 ml of water and administered anally after a bowel movement once per day at approximately 39°C. This treatment is to be suspended during the menses itself.

Along with both the orally and anally administered medicinals, this protocol also uses a topical administration of medicinals on the lower abdomen. Bei Run-pu says to use either *Qi Li San* or *She Xiang Hu Hu Gao* placed over both sides of the lower abdomen. Each application should be left in place for 2 days. Apply for 4 days and then rest for 2 days before reapplying again. The administration of medicinals topically and anally raises the efficacy rate compared to the preceding protocol by another 20%. Thus this approach seems to be superior to either of the two above.

It is interesting to note in the light of the following journal abstract that of the 150 cases of blocked fallopian tubes treated in this protocol, 36 were due to endometriosis, 27 to ovarian cysts, 23 to chronic PID, 29 to post surgery pelvic adhesions, 3 to fallopian tube tuberculosis, and 32 to unknown causes.

6. Sui Song-ling's Protocol[6]

This protocol uses both internally administered decoctions combined with externally applied hot compresses for the treatment of fallopian tube blockage based on the principles of quickening the blood and transforming stasis. The external application of *Xiao Zheng San* was also based on the principle of dispersing concretions. In addition, the internally administered medicinals were modified based on pattern discrimination and also the phases of the menstrual cycle.

The 87 women treated ranged in age from 21-36 years of age. Their condition had lasted from 1 year 7 months to 10 years. Thirty-nine suffered from primary onset infertility and 48 from secondary onset infertility. Most of the cases of secondary onset infertility were associated with post-abortion or postpartum pelvic infections. Among these, 17 women had bilateral adnexitis, 14 one-sided adnexitis, 6 chronic pelvic inflammatory disease, 5 cervical ectropion, and 3 presented with no obvious inflammation. Of the 39 women with primary onset infertility, 18 had bilateral adnexitis, 10 one-sided adnexitis, 7 chronic pelvic inflammatory disease, 2 ovarian cysts, and 2 fallopian tube tuberculosis.

Rx:

1. Internally administered, blood-quickening, stasis-transforming decoction

Rhizoma Smilacis Glabrae (*Tu Fu Ling*)
Ramulus Cinnamomi (*Gui Zhi*)
Semen Pruni Persicae (*Tao Ren*)

---

6   Sui Song-ling, "Clinical Experiences in the Treatment of 87 Cases of Fallopian Tube Blockage with Internally Administered and Externally Applied Medicinals," *He Nan Zhong Yi (Henan Traditional Chinese Medicine)*, No. 1, 1993, p. 23-24

Radix Rubrus Paeoniae Lactiflorae (*Chi Shao*)
Radix Salviae Miltiorrhizae (*Dan Shen*)
Rhizoma Praeparata Cyperi Rotundi (*Zhi Xiang Fu*)
Squama Manitis (*Chuan Shan Jia*)
Semen Vaccariae Segetalis (*Wang Bu Liu Xing*)
Lang Mu (狼目)

Additions & subtractions based on pattern discrimination: If there is simultaneous scorching lower abdominal heat, piercing pain, and yellow abnormal vaginal discharge, delete Ramulus Cinnamomi and add Caulis Sargentodoxae (*Hong Teng*), Radix Scutellariae Barbatae (*Ban Zhi Lian*), Flos Lonicerae Japonicae (*Yin Hua*), Fructus Forsythiae Suspensae (*Lian Qiao*), and Semen Benincasae Hispidae (*Dong Gua Ren*). If there is chilly lower abdominal pain, fear of chill, and the tongue has static spots, add Rhizoma Corydalis Yanhusuo (*Yuan Hu*), Radix Linderae Strychnifoliae (*Wu Yao*), Fructus Evodiae Rutecarpae (*Wu Zhu Yu*), Rhizoma Sparganii (*San Leng*), Rhizoma Curcumae Zedoariae (*E Zhu*), and Feces Trogopterori Seu Pteromi (*Wu Ling Zhi*). If there is chest oppression and breast distention and pain, add Fructus Citri Sacrodactylis (*Fo Shou*), Tuber Curcumae (*Yu Jin*), Fructus Citri Seu Ponciri (*Zhi Ke*), Fructus Meliae Toosendanis (*Chuan Lian Zi*), and Semen Citri (*Ju He*). If the body is fat with excessive phlegm, add Rhizoma Pinelliae Ternatae (*Ban Xia*), Bulbus Fritillariae Thunbergii (*Bei Mu*), Pericarpium Citri Erythrocarpae (*Ju Hong*), Rhizoma Atractylodis (*Cang Zhu*), and Fructus Crataegi (*Shan Zha*). If there is dizziness and the essence spirit is exhausted and weary, add Radix Codonopsis Pilosulae (*Dang Shen*) and Radix Astragali Membranacei (*Huang Qi*).

2. Externally applied, concretion-dispersing powder

Radix Angelicae Dahuricae (*Du Huo*)
Herba Tougucao (*Tou Gu Cao*)
Sanguis Draconis (*Xue Jie*)
Gummum Olibani (*Ru Xiang*)

Myrrha (*Mo Yao*)
Radix Ledebouriellae Sesloidis (*Fang Feng*)
Flos Carthami Tinctorii (*Hong Hua*)
Eupolyphagae Seu Opisthoplatiae (*Tu Bie Chong*)
Apex Radicis Angelicae Sinensis (*Gui Wei*)
Radix Rubrus Paeoniae Lactiflorae (*Chi Shao*)
Folium Artemesiae Argyii (*Ai Ye*)
Cortex Radicis Acanthopanacis (*Wu Jia Pi*)
Radix Angelicae (*Bai Zhi*)
Fructus Zanthoxyli Bungeani (*Chuan Jia*)

Grind the above herbs into a fine powder, divide and reserve one half in a container for later use. Apply the powder as a hot compress to the lower abdomen or both sides of the lower abdomen. Apply 1-2 times per day for 20-30 minutes each time. One *bao* or packet of herbs can be used for 10 days.

This combined treatment should not be carried out the same way throughout the menstrual cycle. Based on this principle, one should stop using the basic formula and hot compresses during the period itself. According to a discrimination of patterns of the viscera and bowels and vacuity and repletion, if the amount of the menses is scant due to blood vacuity, use *Ba Zhen Tang* with additions and subtractions. If the blood is static, use *Tao Hong Si Wu Tang* with additions and subtractions. If the kidneys are vacuous and the essence blood is insufficient, use *Gui Shen Tang* with additions and subtractions each cycle, 3-5 *ji*, beginning 3-5 days after the cessation of the period.

If, during treatment, one discovers that the patient suffers from painful periods, their hyperthermic BBT curve fluctuates widely, or they present with a monophasic BBT, it is alright to elect to enrich and supplement the liver and kidneys and warm and supplement kidney yang. If there is simultaneous liver depression, one can course the liver and resolve depression. During ovulation, one should warm the *jing* (channels/menses) and open the connecting vessels to promote ovulation in order to disinhibit the ovum's ability to unite with the sperm in the uterus.

If both tubes are completely obstructed, it is alright not to modify the basic decoction for the pattern. In that case, after the period, administer *Ding Kun Dan*, 3-5 pills, or *Liu Wei Di Huang Wan* for 7-10 days. Before the period, add *Quan Lu Wan* or *Wu Ji Bai Feng Wan*. The types of Chinese patent medicine have the ability to regulate the menses and strengthen the corpus luteum function as well as raise the organism's ability to resist disease. It is also acceptable to shorten or lengthen the course of treatment if there is no result.

Sui gives the following criteria for grading the results from this therapy. Cure: Relief of dysmenorrhea, histosalpingogram shows both fallopian tubes open and unobstructed, or the woman conceived during treatment. Improved: Both or one tube partially open and patent, obstruction reduced, and lower abdominal distention and pain lessened. No result: Both fallopian tubes not open. Based on these criteria, the results of this study were that 70 cases were cured, 7 cases improved, and 10 women experienced no result. Thus the total amelioration rate was 80.46%.

Sui also says that, in TCM, this condition corresponds to the traditional Chinese disease categories of *wu zi*, no child, *jue hou*, severed posterity, *dai xia*, abnormal vaginal discharge, *zheng jia*, concretions and conglomerations, *yue jing bu tiao*, menstrual irregularity, etc. According to Sui, this disease is mostly caused by blood vacuity, liver depression, phlegm dampness, and blood stasis. In order to remedy this condition, internal medicinals are not sufficient.

7

Polycystic Ovarian Syndrome

Polycystic ovarian syndrome (PCO), also known as Stein-Leventhal syndrome, is one of a heterogenous group of disorders with great clinical and biochemical variability in which chronic anovulation, because of inappropriate feedback signals to the hypothalamic-pituitary unit, appears to be the common denominator. Typically, patients present with amenorrhea, hirsutism, and obesity. However, patients may instead complain of irregular, profuse uterine bleeding and not exhibit any evidence of excessive pilosity. Commonly, this condition begins at puberty and worsens with age. Patients may present with either primary or secondary amenorrhea.

1. Zhang En-qin *et al.*'s Protocol[1]

In Zhang En-qin *et al.*'s *Zhong Yi Lin Chuang Ge Ke (Various Clinical Specialties in Traditional Chinese Medicine)*, their *fu ke* section includes a discussion of polycystic ovarian syndrome. According to Zhang *et al.*, besides scanty menstruation or amenorrhea, pilosity, obesity, and infertility, women suffering from polycystic ovaries also typically have high serum levels of testosterone and LH but low FSH. Zhang *et al.* divide this condition into two main patterns.

---

[1] Zhang En-qin, *et al.*, *Zhong Yi Lin Chuang Ge Ke (Various Specialties in Traditional Chinese Medicine Vol. I)*, Shanghai College of TCM Press, Shanghai, 1990, p. 254-258

Phlegm Dampness

Pathognomonic manifestations: Amenorrhea or infrequent periods, obesity, excessive hair, a pale, fat tongue with a slimy, white coating, and a deep, relaxed/retarded pulse

Therapeutic principles: Break up phlegm and eliminate dampness, quicken the blood and move stagnation

Rx: *Cang Fu Dao Tan Wan Jia Jian*

Rhizoma Atractylodis (*Cang Zhu*)
Rhizoma Cyperi Rotundi (*Xiang Fu*)
Pericarpium Citri Reticulatae (*Chen Pi*)
processed Rhizoma Pinelliae Ternatae (*Ban Xia*)
Thallus Algae (*Kun Bu*)
Spica Prunellae Vulgaris (*Xia Gu Cao*)
Bulbus Fritillariae (*Bei Mu*)
Squama Manitis (*Chuan Shan Jia*)
Bulbus Pleionis (*Shan Ci Gu*)
Spina Gleditschiae (*Jiao Ci*)
Fructus Citri Seu Ponciri (*Zhi Ke*)
Sclerotium Poriae Cocoris (*Fu Ling*)

Kidney Vacuity

Pathognomonic manifestations: Infrequent, scanty menstruation or amenorrhea, emaciation, excessive hair, low back soreness, dizziness, dislike of cold, loose stools, a pale tongue with a thin, white coating, and a deep, thready pulse

Therapeutic principles: Warm the kidneys, boost the *jing* essence, and scatter nodulation

Rx: *Zuo Gui Wan Jia Jian*

prepared Radix Rehmanniae (*Shu Di*)
Gelatinum Cornu Cervi (*Lu Jiao Jiao*)
Semen Cuscutae (*Tu Si Zi*)
Fructus Rubi (*Fu Pen Zi*)
Rhizoma Cibotii (*Gou Ji*)
Semen Trigonellae Foeni-graeci (*Hu Lu Ba*)
Herba Epimedii (*Xian Ling Pi*)
Rhizoma Polygonati (*Huang Jing*)
Spica Prunellae Vulgaris (*Xia Gu Cao*)

2. Yu Huang's Protocol #1[2]

This protocol reiterates that the two main TCM mechanisms involved in *duo nang luan chao zeng he zheng* or polycystic ovarian syndrome are kidney yang vacuity and phlegm nodulation. Therefore, Yu gives a single guiding formula which takes both these patterns into account with modifications. Hu Xi-ming, in his preface to this protocol, says that, in the case of polycystic ovarian syndrome, the kidneys are vacuous and phlegm is replete. He explains the relationship between the kidneys and phlegm by stating that, if the kidneys are vacuous, they are not able to drain and vacate fluids and humors from the lower burner. These then may stagnate and congeal. In addition, Hu points out that, because the liver and kidneys share a common, source, kidney insufficiency may cause or aggravate any tendency to liver depression. If this depression is chronic or severe, it can transform into fire and damage yin. In addition, either stagnant qi or stagnant fluids can, over time, give rise to blood stasis. Therefore, according to Hu, the main disease mechanisms and patterns involved with polycystic ovarian syndrome are kidney vacuity, either yin or yang vacuity, liver depression, phlegm dampness, and blood stasis.

---

[2]   Hu Xi-ming, *op. cit.*, p. 159-161

Rx: *Yu Shi Wen Bu Fang*

prepared Radix Rehmanniae (*Shu Di*)
Rhizoma Polygonati (*Huang Jing*)
Herba Epimedii (*Xian Ling Pi*)
Fructus Psoraleae Corylifoliae (*Bu Gu Zhi*)
Squama Manitis (*Shan Jia*)
Spina Gleditschiae Sinensis (*Zao Jiao Ci*)
Bing Qiu Zi (冰球子)
Bulbus Fritillariae (*Bei Mu*)

Additions & subtractions based on pattern discrimination: If there is fear of chill, add Radix Praeparatus Aconiti Carmichaeli (*Fu Zi*) and Cortex Cinnamomi (*Rou Gui*). For liver depression, add Cortex Radicis Moutan (*Dan Pi*), Fructus Praeparatus Gardeniae Jasminoidis (*Chao Shan Zhi*), Radix Bupleuri (*Chai Hu*), Radix Angelicae Sinensis (*Dang Gui*), and Pericarpium Viridis Citri Reticulatae (*Qing Pi*), and delete Spina Gleditschiae, *Bing Qiu Zi*, and Bulbus Fritillariae.

Of 133 women treated with this protocol, 82.7% did ovulate. Of the 76 women complaining of infertility, 36 conceived.

3. Yu Huang's Protocol #2[3]

This protocol uses four different formulas for each of the four phases of the menstrual cycle. Further, women are categorized into kidney yang insufficiency types and kidney yin insufficiency types with each group receiving their own formulas.

---

[3]   *Ibid.*, p. 161-162

Phase I

Rx: *Cu Luan Bao Tang*

If there is kidney yang insufficiency, use:

Rhizoma Curculiginis Orchoidis (*Xian Mao*)
Herba Epimedii (*Xian Ling Pi*)
Radix Angelicae Sinensis (*Dang Gui*)
Radix Dioscoreae Oppositae (*Shan Yao*)
Semen Cuscutae (*Tu Si Zi*)
Radix Morindae Officinalis (*Ba Ji Rou*)
Herba Cistanchis (*Rou Cong Rong*)
prepared Radix Rehmanniae (*Shu Di*)

If there is kidney yin insufficiency, use:

Fructus Ligustri Lucidi (*Nu Zhen Zi*)
Herba Ecliptae Prostratae (*Han Lian Cao*)
Radix Salviae Miltiorrhizae (*Dan Shen*)
Radix Dioscoreae Oppositae (*Shan Yao*)
Semen Cuscutae (*Tu Si Zi*)
prepared Radix Rehmanniae (*Shu Di*)
Herba Cistanchis (*Rou Cong Rong*)
Radix Praeparatus Polygoni Multiflori (*Zhi Shou Wu*)

Phase II

Rx: *Cu Pai Luan Tang*

If there is kidney yang insufficiency, use:

Radix Angelicae Sinensis (*Dang Gui*)
Radix Salviae Miltiorrhizae (*Dan Shen*)
Semen Leonuri Heterophylli (*Chong Wei Zi*)

Semen Pruni Persicae (*Tao Ren*)
Flos Carthami Tinctorii (*Hong Hua*)
Caulis Millettiae Seu Spatholobi (*Ji Xue Teng*)
Radix Dipsaci (*Xu Duan*)
Rhizoma Cyperi Rotundi (*Xiang Fu*)
Ramulus Cinnamomi (*Gui Zhi*)

If there is kidney yin insufficiency, use:

Radix Salviae Miltiorrhizae (*Dan Shen*)
Radix Rubrus Paeoniae Lactiflorae (*Chi Shao*)
Herba Lycopi Lucidi (*Ze Lan*)
prepared Radix Rehmanniae (*Shu Di*)
Fructus Lycii Chinensis (*Gou Qi Zi*)
Semen Pruni Persicae (*Tao Ren*)
Flos Carthami Tinctorii (*Hong Hua*)
Semen Coicis Lachryma-jobi (*Yi Ren*)
Rhizoma Cyperi Rotundi (*Xiang Fu*)

Phase III

Rx: *Cu Huang Ti Tang*

If there is kidney yang insufficiency, use:

Gelatinum Corii Asini (*E Jiao*)
Plastrum Testudinis (*Gui Ban*)
Radix Angelicae Sinensis (*Dang Gui*)
prepared Radix Rehmanniae (*Shu Di*)
Radix Polygoni Multiflori (*Shou Wu*)
Semen Cuscutae (*Tu Si Zi*)
Radix Dipsaci (*Xu Duan*)
Rhizoma Cyperi Rotundi (*Xiang Fu*)
Ramulus Cinnamomi (*Gui Zhi*)

180

If there is kidney yin insufficiency, use:

Radix Salviae Miltiorrhizae (*Dan Shen*)
Plastrum Testudinis (*Gui Ban*)
Fructus Lycii Chinensis (*Gou Qi Zi*)
Fructus Ligustri Lucidi (*Nu Zhen Zi*)
Herba Ecliptae Prostratae (*Han Lian Cao*)
prepared Radix Rehmanniae (*Shu Di*)
processed Radix Polygoni Multiflori (*Shou Wu*)
Herba Cistanchis (*Rou Cong Rong*)
Semen Cuscutae (*Tu Si Zi*)

Phase IV

Rx: *Huo Xue Tiao Jing Tang*

If there is kidney yang insufficiency, use:

Radix Angelicae Sinensis (*Dang Gui*)
prepared Radix Rehmanniae (*Shu Di*)
Radix Salviae Miltiorrhizae (*Dan Shen*)
Radix Rubrus Paeoniae Lactiflorae (*Chi Shao*)
Herba Lycopi Lucidi (*Ze Lan*)
Rhizoma Ligustici Wallichii (*Chuan Xiong*)
Rhizoma Cyperi Rotundi (*Xiang Fu*)
Semen Leonuri Heterophylli (*Chong Wei Zi*)

If there is kidney yin insufficiency, use:

Radix Salviae Miltiorrhizae (*Dan Shen*)
Radix Rubrus Paeoniae Lactiflorae (*Chi Shao*)
Herba Lycopi Lucidi (*Ze Lan*)
prepared Radix Rehmanniae (*Shu Di*)
Sclerotium Poriae Cocoris (*Fu Ling*)
Semen Leonuri Heterophylli (*Chong Wei Zi*)

Radix Angelicae Sinensis (*Dang Gui*)
Rhizoma Cyperi Rotundi (*Xiang Fu*)

Twenty-seven cases were treated with this protocol and after 3 whole months all ovulated. Twenty-four of these women conceived within 3 years of this protocol for a success rate of 88.8%.

Unlike the above protocol, there is no attention to phlegm nodulation given in this treatment. However, one of the things I like about this protocol is that it does give separate formulas for those who either are predominantly kidney yin or yang vacuous. These formulas may be used as hints for modifying other protocols in this book, such as Sun Ning-quan's for luteal phase defect. In that protocol, Sun Ning-quan does not, from my opinion, differentiate enough between yin and yang vacuities. Especially during midcycle, when yin vacuity and flaring of yang fire often occur, Sun's protocol may be too hot and provoke hot symptoms such as midcycle bleeding. Lin, however, gives an ovulatory formula for those with more prominent yin vacuity which quickens the blood but does not warm the uterus. Thus it is useful to compare phased protocols even under different diseases to get a better idea of how to tailor a protocol to an individual patient's personal pattern.

4. Yu Huang's Protocol for Galactorrhea-amenorrhea Syndrome[4]

Some women with polycystic ovarian syndrome, estrogen deficiency, or luteal phase defect may have a combination of galactorrhea and amenorrhea. From a Western point of view, this is mostly due to microadenomas of the pituitary causing excessive quantities of prolactin (PR). Below is a protocol by the same Master Yu as above describing his treatment of two cases of this syndrome.

---

[4]   *Ibid.*, p. 163-165

Yu's assumption is that this condition is primarily associated with liver heat and depression combined with kidney vacuity. Since the liver channel sends an internal branch to the nipple and since heat can force various fluids out of the body, Yu sees galactorrhea as a liver depression, transformative fire condition, while he relates the amenorrhea more to kidney vacuity.

Rx: *Qing Gan Bu Shen Tang*

Cortex Radicis Moutan (*Dan Pi*)
stir-fried Fructus Gardeniae Jasminoidis (*Shan Zhi*)
Radix Bupleuri (*Chai Hu*)
Radix Angelicae Sinensis (*Dang Gui*)
Pericarpium Viridis Citri Reticulatae (*Qing Pi*)
Radix Rehmanniae (*Sheng Di*)
Rhizoma Polygonati (*Huang Jing*)
Herba Epimedii (*Xian Ling Pi*)
Fructus Psoraleae Corylifoliae (*Bu Gu Zhi*)
Squama Manitis (*Shan Jia*)

Yu says that in clinical practice, even better results can be obtained by combining this formula with *Sheng Mai Ya Tang*. This is composed of 100-200g of Fructus Germinatus Hordei Vulgaris. This ingredient is an empirical specific for stopping lactation.

8

Endometriosis

Endometriosis is another Western gynecological disease category associated with infertility. It is the proliferation and cyclic growth of endometrial tissue outside of the endometrium. Modern Western medicine is not yet sure of the exact mechanisms at work and why some women develop endometriosis. It is assumed that it is a hormonal dyscrasia. Recent Chinese research suggests that this hormonal imbalance may be due to autoimmune ovaritis. I discuss such ovaritis in Chapter 10 on candidiasis below.

Based on my own clinical experience in treating this condition, the best Chinese discussion of it I have seen to date is by Cao Ling-xian and Tang Ji-fu. I have, however, supplemented Cao and Tang's discussion by adding some formulas from Zhang En-qin *et al.* in order to give practitioners more options.

1. Cao & Tang's Protocol[1]

Cao and Tang posit four main patterns associated with endometriosis. These are:

---

[1] Cao Ling-Xian & Tang Ji-fu, "Endometriosis as Treated by Traditional Chinese Medicine," translated by C.S. Cheung & Carolyn Atkinson, *Journal of American College of TCM*, No. 1, 1983, p. 57

1. Qi stagnation, blood stasis

Cao and Tang recognize that in the case of this pattern, there may be either more qi stagnation and less blood stasis or more blood stasis and less qi stagnation. Depending upon which is prominent, they give two guiding formulas.

Rx: *Si Ni San*

Radix Bupleuri (*Chai Hu*)
Fructus Citri Seu Ponciri (*Zhi Ke*)
Radix Albus Paeoniae Lactiflorae (*Bai Shao*)
Radix Glycyrrhizae (*Gan Cao*)

This is the guiding formula which Cao and Tang recommend for more pronounced qi stagnation endometriosis. This then is to be modified for the individual's unique presentation. It should be remembered that *Xiao Yao San* is believed to be a modification of this formula and, therefore, one's scope should not be too narrow in modifying this base prescription.

Tao Hong Si Wu Tang

Semen Pruni Persicae (*Tao Ren*)
Flos Carthami Tinctorii (*Hong Hua*)
prepared Radix Rehmanniae (*Shu Di*)
Radix Rubrus Paeoniae Lactiflorae (*Chi Shao*)
Radix Angelicae Sinensis (*Dang Gui*)
Rhizoma Ligustici Wallichii (*Chuan Xiong*)

Additions & subtractions based on pattern discrimination: If there is intense pain in the lower abdomen, add Fructus Zanthoxyli Bungeani (*Chua Jiao*), Fructus Foeniculi Vulgaris (*Xiao Hui Xiang*), Feces Trogopterori Seu Pteromi (*Wu Ling Zhi*), and Pollen Typhae (*Pu Huang*). If there are blood clots in the menstruate, add Rhizoma

186

Sparganii (*San Leng*), and Rhizoma Curcumae Zedoariae (*E Zhu*). If there is stasis and heat with constipation, add Radix Et Rhizoma Rhei (*Da Huang*), and Mirabilitum (*Mang Xiao*). If the condition is chronic and blood stasis has entered the *luo mai*, add Buthus Martensi (*Quan Xie*) and Eupolyphagae Seu Opisthoplatiae (*Tu Bie Chong*) etc.

Zhang En-qin *et al.* give the following formula for the treatment of endometriosis due to qi stagnation, blood stasis. It is a modification of *Shao Fu Zhu Yu Tang* discussed by Cao and Tang below under the next pattern.

Tong Jing Fang

Radix Angelicae Sinensis (*Dang Gui*)
Rhizoma Ligustici Wallichii (*Chuan Xiong*)
Radix Salviae Miltiorrhizae (*Dan Shen*)
Radix Cyathulae (*Niu Xi*)
Radix Rubrus Paeoniae Lactiflorae (*Chi Shao*)
Ramulus Cinnamomi (*Gui Zhi*)
Rhizoma Cyperi Rotundi (*Xiang Fu*)
Rhizoma Corydalis Yanhusuo (*Yuan Hu*)
Sanguis Draconis (*Xue Jie*)
Myrrha (*Mo Yao*)
Feces Trogopterori Seu Pteromi (*Wu Ling Zhi*)
Pollen Typhae (*Pu Huang*)

2. Accumulation of cold, blood stasis

Rx: Shao Fu Zhu Yu Tang

Radix Angelicae Sinensis (*Dang Gui*)
Radix Rubrus Paeoniae Lactiflorae (*Chi Shao*)
Rhizoma Ligustici Wallichii (*Chuan Xiong*)
dry Rhizoma Zingiberis (*Gan Jiang*)
Cortex Cinnamomi (*Rou Gui*)

Pollen Typhae (*Pu Huang*)
Feces Trogopterori Seu Pteromi (*Wu Ling Zhi*)
Rhizoma Corydalis Yanhusuo (*Yan Hu*)
Fructus Foeniculi Vulgaris (*Xiao Hui Xiang*)
Myrrha (*Mo Yao*)

Additions & subtractions based on pattern discrimination: If there is intense pain with very cold limbs, perspiration, and a cold appearance, add Radix Praeparatus Aconiti Carmichaeli (*Fu Zi*) and Radix Aconiti (*Wu Tou*). If there is cold dampness, add Radix Et Rhizoma Notopterygii (*Qiang Huo*) and Radix Angelicae Duhuo (*Du Huo*). If there is nausea and vomiting, add Fructus Evodiae Rutecarpae (*Wu Zhu Yu*). If there is diarrhea, add Semen Trigonellae Foeni-graeci (*Hu Lu Ba*) and Fructus Psoraleae Corylifoliae (*Bu Gu Zhi*).

This formula is for replete cold causing blood stasis and stagnation in the lower burner.

San Jie Fang

stir-fried Radix Angelicae Sinensis (*Dang Gui*)
Radix Salviae Miltiorrhizae (*Dan Shen*)
Radix Rubrus Paeoniae Lactiflorae (*Chi Shao*)
Radix Cyathulae (*Chuan Niu Xi*)
processed Rhizoma Cyperi Rotundi (*Xiang Fu*)
Ramulus Cinnamomi (*Gui Zhi*)
Herba Sargassi (*Hai Zao*)
mix-fried Squama Manitis (*Chuan Shan Jia*)
Spina Gleditschiae (*Jiao Ci*)
Sanguis Draconis (*Xue Jie*)
Rhizoma Curcumae Zedoariae (*E Zhu*)

This formula is given by Zhang En-qin *et al*.

Wen Jing Tang

Radix Angelicae Sinensis (*Dang Gui*)
Radix Albus Paeoniae Lactiflorae (*Bai Shao*)
Rhizoma Ligustici Wallichii (*Chuan Xiong*)
Cortex Radicis Moutan (*Dan Pi*)
Gelatinum Corii Asini (*E Jiao*)
Ramulus Cinnamomi (*Gui Zhi*)
Fructus Evodiae Rutecarpae (*Wu Zhu Yu*)
Tuber Ophiopogonis Japonicae (*Mai Dong*)
Radix Panacis Ginseng (*Ren Shen*)
Rhizoma Pinelliae Ternatae (*Ban Xia*)
fresh Rhizoma Zingiberis (*Sheng Jiang*)
Radix Glycyrrhizae (*Gan Cao*)

This formula is recommended by Cao and Tang for vacuity cold of the *chong* and *ren* with blood stasis.

Additions & subtractions based on pattern discrimination: If lower abdominal cold pain is more severe, delete Tuber Ophiopogonis Japonicae and Cortex Radicis Moutan, substitute Cortex Cinnamomi (*Rou Gui*) for Ramulus Cinnamomi, and add Fructus Foeniculi Vulgaris (*Xiao Hui Xiang*) and Folium Artemesiae Argyii (*Ai Ye*). If qi stagnation is pronounced, add Rhizoma Cyperi Rotundi (*Xiang Fu*) and Radix Linderae Strychnifoliae (*Wu Yao*). If there is qi vacuity, add Radix Astragali Membranacei (*Huang Qi*). For infertility due to blood vacuity and cold, add Pericarpium Viridis Citri Reticulatae (*Qing Pi*) and Rhizoma Cyperi Rotundi (*Xiang Fu*). For chronic endometriosis, add Gummum Olibani (*Ru Xiang*) and Myrrha (*Mo Yao*).

3. Accumulation of heat, blood stasis

Rx: *Xiao Chai Hu Tang He Gui Zhi Tang*

Radix Bupleuri (*Chai Hu*)

Radix Albus Paeoniae Lactiflorae (*Bai Shao*)
Ramulus Cinnamomi (*Gui Zhi*)
Radix Scutellariae Baicalensis (*Huang Qin*)
Rhizoma Pinelliae Ternatae (*Ban Xia*)
Radix Codonopsis Pilosulae (*Dang Shen*)
mix-fried Radix Glycyrrhizae (*Zhi Gan Cao*)
fresh Rhizoma Zingiberis (*Sheng Jiang*)
Fructus Zizyphi Jujubae (*Da Zao*)

Cao and Tang say to use this formula if there is abdominal pain with the arrival of the menses accompanied by fever. This formula is another possible one for use with *yu re* or stasis heat discussed above.

Tao He Cheng Qi Tang

Semen Pruni Persicae (*Tao Ren*)
Ramulus Cinnamomi (*Gui Zhi*)
Radix Et Rhizoma Rhei (*Da Huang*)
Mirabilitum (*Mang Xiao*)
mix-fried Radix Glycyrrhizae (*Zhi Gan Cao*)

Cao and Tang suggest this formula for abdominal pain with replete heat in the stomach and intestines and constipation.

Additions & subtractions based on pattern discrimination: If there is menstrual irregularity and painful periods, add Radix Angelicae Sinensis (*Dang Gui*) and Flos Carthami Tinctorii (*Hong Hua*). If qi stagnation is pronounced, add Rhizoma Cyperi Rotundi (*Xiang Fu*) and Pericarpium Viridis Citri Reticulatae (*Qing Pi*). If blood stasis is severe, add Radix Rubrus Paeoniae Lactiflorae (*Chi Shao*) and Radix Pseudoginseng (*San Qi*). If there is premenstrual nosebleed and the blood is purple and clotty, add Radix Rehmanniae (*Sheng Di*) and Rhizoma Imperatae Cylindricae (*Bai Mao Geng*).

Wu Mei Wan

Fructus Pruni Mume (*Wu Mei*)
Herba Cum Radice Asari Sieboldi (*Xi Xin*)
dry Rhizoma Zingiberis (*Gan Jiang*)
Fructus Zanthoxyli Bungeani (*Chuan Jiao*)
Ramulus Cinnamomi (*Gui Zhi*)
Radix Praeparatus Aconiti Carmichaeli (*Fu Zi*)
Cortex Phellodendri (*Huang Bai*)
Rhizoma Coptidis Chinensis (*Huang Lian*)
Radix Angelicae Sinensis (*Dang Gui*)
Radix Codonopsis Pilosulae (*Dang Shen*)

Cao and Tang recommend this formula for chronic, intractable dysmenorrhea with a combination of hot and cold, repletion and vacuity. I have found this formula to be brilliantly effective in the right cases and I will discuss this further under candidiasis below. The reader should remember that the heat in *yu re* is damp heat.

Additions & subtractions based on pattern discrimination: If there are no cold symptoms, delete Ramulus Cinnamomi and Radix Praeparatus Aconiti Carmichaeli. If the righteous qi has not yet been damaged, delete Radix Codonopsis Pilosulae and Radix Angelicae Sinensis. If there is severe abdominal pain, add Fructus Meliae Toosendanis (*Chuan Lian Zi*) and Radix Saussureae Seu Vladimiriae (*Mu Xiang*). If there is constipation, add Semen Arecae Catechu (*Bing Lang*) and Fructus Immaturus Citri Seu Ponciri (*Zhi Shi*). If there is nausea and vomiting, add Fructus Evodiae Rutecarpae (*Wu Zhu Yu*) and Rhizoma Pinelliae Ternatae (*Ban Xia*). If there are loose stools with the period, add Radix Saussureae Seu Vladimiriae (*Mu Xiang*) and Radix Albus Paeoniae Lactiflorae (*Bai Shao*).

4. Qi and blood vacuity, blood stasis

Cao and Tang say that if there is qi vacuity, it may be impossible to remove blood stasis by attacking methods alone. This will only make the qi more vacuous and the stasis will persist without improvement. Therefore, when qi vacuity complicates blood stasis, one should boost the qi and move the qi, quicken the blood and transform stasis. Cao and Tang give four guiding formulas for this purpose.

Rx: *Huang Qi Jian Zhong Tang*

Radix Astragali Membranacei (*Huang Qi*)
Maltose (*Yi Tang*)
Ramulus Cinnamomi (*Gui Zhi*)
Radix Albus Paeoniae Lactiflorae (*Bai Shao*)
mix-fried Radix Glycyrrhizae (*Zhi Gan Cao*)
fresh Rhizoma Zingiberis (*Sheng Jiang*)
Fructus Zizyphi Jujubae (*Da Zao*)

This formula is for use when qi vacuity predominates over blood vacuity.

Dang Gui Jian Zhong Tang

Radix Angelicae Sinensis (*Dang Gui*)
Maltose (*Yi Tang*)
Ramulus Cinnamomi (*Gui Zhi*)
Radix Albus Paeoniae Lactiflorae (*Bai Shao*)
fresh Rhizoma Zingiberis (*Sheng Jiang*)
Fructus Zizyphi Jujubae (*Da Zao*)
mix-fried Radix Glycyrrhizae (*Zhi Gan Cao*)

This formula is for use when blood vacuity predominates over qi vacuity.

Fu Zi Li Zhong Wan

Radix Praeparatus Aconiti Carmichaeli (*Fu Zi*)
dry Rhizoma Zingiberis (*Gan Jiang*)
Radix Panacis Ginseng (*Ren Shen*)

Rhizoma Atractylodis Macrocephalae (*Bai Zhu*)
Radix Praeparatus Glycyrrhizae (*Zhi Gan Cao*)

This formula is for use when vacuity is complicated by cold.

Bu Zhong Yi Qi Tang

Radix Astragali Membranacei (*Huang Qi*)
Radix Codonopsis Pilosulae (*Dang Shen*)
mix-fried Radix Glycyrrhizae (*Zhi Gan Cao*)
Rhizoma Atractylodis Macrocephalae (*Bai Zhu*)
Radix Angelicae Sinensis (*Dang Gui*)
Radix Bupleuri (*Chai Hu*)
Rhizoma Cimicifugae (*Sheng Ma*)
Pericarpium Citri Reticulatae (*Chen Pi*)

Cao and Tang say to select this formula if there is qi vacuity fever during menstruation.

For the treatment of endometriosis, medicinals for quickening the blood and transforming stasis can be added to any of the above four formulas as appropriate.

To these four patterns, we may add another from Zhang En-qin *et al.*:

5. Kidney vacuity, blood stasis

Rx: Xue Beng Fang

stir-fried Radix Angelicae Sinensis (*Dang Gui*)
Pollen Typhae (*Sheng Pu Huang*)
Radix Achyranthis Bidentatae (*Huai Niu Xi*)
Radix Salviae Miltiorrhizae (*Dan Shen*)
Radix Albus Paeoniae Lactiflorae (*Bai Shao*)
Radix Rubrus Paeoniae Lactiflorae (*Chi Shao*)

processed Rhizoma Cyperi Rotundi (*Xiang Fu*)
Dolomitum (*Hua Rui Shi*)
prepared and carbonized Radix Et Rhizoma Rhei (*Jun Tan*)
Sanguis Draconis (*Xue Jie*)

Additions & subtractions based on pattern discrimination: If there is no excessive bleeding, delete Dolomitum. If there is damp heat combined with kidney vacuity evidenced by a red tongue with slimy, yellow coating, a thready, floating pulse in the left *chi* but a deep, slippery pulse in the right *chi*, low back and upper medial thigh pain, chilled extremities, and frequent urination, use regular Radix Et Rhizoma Rhei (*Da Huang*) instead of carbonized Radix Et Rhizoma Rhei along with other appropriate modifications. This can be a confusing pattern. In clinical practice, I have occasionally combined the above formula with *Tao He Cheng Qi Tang* with additions and subtractions to also treat this complicated pattern of mixed vacuity and repletion.

2. Luo Jian-hua's Protocol[2]

This very recently published protocol for the treatment of endometriosis continues to assume that blood stasis is the primary disease mechanism involved in endometriosis. Luo says that endometriosis is characterized by blood stasis and knotting in the lower abdomen affecting the two vessels, the *chong* and *ren*. Qi and blood transportation and movement are not easy and lack of free flow leads to pain. The main principles Luo advances for the treatment of endometriosis are to quicken the blood and transform stasis. Luo then used *Jia Wei Gui Zhi Fu Ling Wan* to accomplish those principles.

At first, the choice of this formula does not look particularly brilliant.

---

[2]   Luo Jian-hua, "*Jia Wei Gui Zhi Fu Ling Wan Zhi Liao Zi Gong Nei Mo Yi Wei Zhong 50 Li* (50 Cases of Endometriosis Treated by Jia Wei Gui Zhi Fu Ling Wan)," *Hu Nan Zhong Yi Za Zhi* (*Hunan Journal of TCM*), No. 6, 1992, p. 30

However, its combination of warm, spicy ingredients with bitter, cold ingredients does inherently address a more complicated scenario than Luo describes. The standard version of this formula treats vacuity cold and blood stasis complicated by heat in the blood level. This heat in the blood level is typically damp heat and this formula does include an ingredient, Sclerotium Poriae Cocoris (*Fu Ling*) which strengthens the spleen, the root of the transportation and transformation of water, and seeps dampness. Luo has modified this formula by adding Radix Et Rhizoma Rhei (*Da Huang*) which not only clears heat from the large intestine but clears and eliminates damp heat, clears heat from the *xue fen*, and quickens the blood and transforms stasis. In addition, this medicinal is also a powerful antifungal.

When the ingredients in this formula are analyzed from this perspective, this formula is seen to be appropriate for treating dampness and heat in the lower burner and intestines, heat entering the blood level, vacuity cold due to intestinal damp heat injuring the source of the transformation and generation of the kidneys, and blood stasis. This is a more complicated scenario than simply blood stasis. It takes into account that candidiasis is commonly present in patients with endometriosis and, as we shall see below, it also, therefore, takes into account autoimmune ovaritis. The various modifications of Luo's guiding formula all suggest the various complications that are typically involved in this condition.

Rx: *Jia Wei Fu Ling Wan*

Ramulus Cinnamomi (*Chuan Gui Zhi*)
Radix Et Rhizoma Rhei (*Da Huang*)
Semen Pruni Persicae (*Tao Ren*)
Sclerotium Poriae Cocoris (*Fu Ling*)
Cortex Radicis Moutan (*Dan Pi*)
Radix Albus Paeoniae Lactiflorae (*Bai Shao*)
Rhizoma Corydalis Yanhusuo (*Yan Hu Suo*)

One *ji* was administered per day decocted in water.

Additions & subtractions based on pattern discrimination: If there were cold extremities with lower abdominal chilling, an ashen white face with purplish lips, a weary spirit and lack of strength, and infertility, all indicating vacuity cold, Fructus Evodiae Rutecarpae (*Wu Zhu Yu*), 6g, and Radix Codonopsis Pilosulae (*Dang Shen*) and Gelatinum Corii Asini (*E Jiao*) were added to supplement vacuity and warm the *jing*.

If the menstrual cycle was short but the amount excessive, indicating evil heat, carbonized Pollen Typhae (*Pu Huang*), processed Rhizoma Cyperi Rotundi (*Xiang Fu*), Radix Salviae Miltiorrhizae (*Dan Shen*), Radix Angelicae Sinensis (*Dang Gui*), Fructus Gardeniae Jasminoidis (*Zhi Zi*), and Pulvis Radicis Pseudoginseng (*San Qi Fen*) were added to clear heat and stop bleeding. These additions make it clear that Luo sees this heat as stagnant heat.

If the menstrual cycle was short and scanty, indicating more serious blood stasis forcing the blood outside its pathway, Pollen Typhae (*Sheng Pu Huang*), Feces Trogopterori (*Wu Ling Zhi*), Fructus Crataegi (*Shan Zha*), Rhizoma Curcumae Zedoariae (*E Zhu*), Radix Achyranthis Bidentatae (*Niu Xi*), Radix Angelicae Sinensis (*Dang Gui*), and Radix Bupleuri (*Chai Hu*), were added to dispel stasis and quicken the blood.

And, if there were lumps inside the abdomen, indicating even more serious blood stasis, Radix Salviae Miltiorrhizae (*Dan Shen*), Squama Manitis (*Chuan Shan Jia*), Herba Sargassi (*Hai Zao*), Rhizoma Ligustici Wallichii (*Chuan Xiong*), Gummum Olibani (*Ru Xiang*), and Myrrha (*Mo Yao*), were added to crack or cleave stasis.

Using this protocol, Luo treated 50 women with endometriosis between the ages of 21-49. Of these 42 were married and 8 were single. Thirty-seven had experienced miscarriage and 34 were infertile. Twenty-three of these women had suffered with their disease for 1-2 years. Twelve had had endometriosis for 2-3 years, and 15 had experienced symptoms for more than 3 years. In addition, 41 women experienced chronic severe dysmenorrhea, while 9 women's pain was of recent onset. Accompanying all these women's menses was a heavy, distended feeling in their low back and abdomen extending to their anus and genitalia. Twenty-seven cases also complained of cold extremities and a chilly feeling in their lower abdomens. And finally, in 41 cases, the menses arrived between days 15-24, and in 9 cases, between days 24-29. In 37 cases, the amount of the menses was excessive, and in 5 cases it was scant. Twenty-nine women had lumps in their pelvic cavities.

Typically, these women's tongues were pale purple or dark red. The tips had purple spots. Their coating was either thin and white or thin and yellow. Underneath the tongue, the blood vessels were distended and greenish purple. These women's pulses tended to be wiry and tight, wiry and fine, or choppy/astringent.

Using the above protocol, 29 cases experienced a complete cure of their symptoms, while the other 21 women experienced obvious improvement. Cure meant that their menses arrived normally, was without pain, that its amount and color were normal, and that the period arrived between 25-30 days. Obvious improvement meant that the women still experienced some slow degree of lower abdominal heaviness and distention. In order to achieve these results, the shortest duration of therapy was 3 whole months or cycles. Most of the women required between 6 and 24 months of treatment. Unfortunately for the purposes of this book, no conception rates were given.

3. Cai Xiao-sun's Protocol[3]

This protocol integrates the treatment of endometriosis with a multi-phased approach specifically for the treatment of infertility due to endometriosis. It combines both the assumption that endometriosis is associated with stasis and stagnation and that infertility is associated

---

[3] Deng Zhen-ming, "Cai Xiao-sun's Experiences Treating Endometriosis," *Zhong Yi Za Zhi (Journal of TCM)*, No. 11, 1991, p. 15-16

with kidney insufficiency. Deng Zhen-ming, the author of the article in which this protocol appears, says that 22-66% of women with endometriosis are infertile.

From the end of menstruation to ovulation, use:

Yun I Fang

Sclerotium Poriae Cocoris (*Yun Fu Ling*)
Folium Photinae Serrulatae (*Shi Nan Ye*)
prepared Radix Rehmanniae (*Shu Di*)
Ramulus Cinnamomi (*Gui Zhi*)
Rhizoma Curculiginis Orchoidis (*Xian Mao*)
Herba Epimedii (*Xian Ling Pi*)
Fructus Liquidambaris Taiwaniae (*Lu Lu Tong*)
Flos Caryophylli (*Gong Ding Xiang*)
Radix Cyathulae (*Chuan Niu Xi*)

plus ### Nei Yi III Fang

Sclerotium Poriae Cocoris (*Yun Fu Ling*)
Ramulus Cinnamomi (*Gui Zhi*)
Semen Pruni Persicae (*Tao Ren*)
Radix Rubrus Paeoniae Lactiflorae (*Chi Shao*)
Cortex Radicis Moutan (*Dan Pi*)
Spina Gleditschiae Chinensis (*Zao Jiao Ci*)
Lignum Suberalatum Euonymi (*Gui Jian Yu*)
Herba Salviae Chinensis (*Shi Jian Chuan*)

It is my assumption that when these two formulas are used together, one does not double the amounts of the duplicate ingredients. This combination is meant to foster the kidneys and open the *luo* or connecting vessels.

After ovulation and to the premenstruum, for 3-7 days, use:

Yun II Fang

prepared Radix Rehmanniae (*Shu Di*)
Radix Rehmanniae (*Sheng Di*)
Sclerotium Poriae Cocoris (*Yun Fu Ling*)
Folium Photinae Serrulatae (*Shi Nan Ye*)
Cornu Degelatinum Cervi (*Lu Jiao Shuang*)
Herba Epimedii (*Xian Ling Pi*)
Radix Morindae Officinalis (*Ba Ji Tian*)
Herba Cistanchis (*Rou Cong Rong*)
Herba Ecliptae Prostratae (*Han Lian Cao*)
Fructus Ligustri Lucidi (*Nu Zhen Zi*)
Radix Achyranthis Bidentatae (*Huai Niu Xi*)

plus *Nei Yi III Fang* above

This combination is meant to foster the kidneys, warm, and heat.

From a few days before the onset of menstruation or in order to stop pain during the period itself, use:

Nei Yi I Fang

Radix Angelicae Sinensis (*Dang Gui*)
Radix Salviae Miltiorrhizae (*Dan Shen*)
Radix Achyranthis Bidentatae (*Niu Xi*)
Radix Rubrus Paeoniae Lactiflorae (*Chi Shao*)
Rhizoma Cyperi Rotundi (*Xiang Fu*)
Rhizoma Ligustici Wallichii (*Chuan Xiong*)
Ramulus Cinnamomi (*Gui Zhi*)
Myrrha (*Mo Yao*)
Feces Trogopterori Seu Pteromi (*Wu Ling Zhi*)
Pollen Typhae (*Pu Huang*)
Sanguis Draconis (*Xue Jie*)

or *Nei Yi II Fang*

Radix Angelicae Sinensis (*Dang Gui*)
Radix Achyranthis Bidentatae (*Niu Xi*)
Radix Rubrus Paeoniae Lactiflorae (*Chi Shao*)
Rhizoma Cyperi Rotundi (*Xiang Fu*)
prepared and carbonized Radix Et Rhizoma Rhei (*Jun*)
Pollen Typhae (*Sheng Pu Huang*)
Radix Salviae Miltiorrhizae (*Dan Shen*)
Dolomitum (*Hua Rui Shi*)
Sanguis Draconis (*Xue Jie*)
Zhen Ling Dan, wrapped separately (see below)

Zhen Ling Dan

Limonitum (*Yu Liang Shi*)
Fluoritum (*Zi Shi Ying*)
Hallyositum Rubrum (*Chi Shi Zhi*)
Haematitum (*Dai Zhe Shi*)
Gummum Olibani (*Ru Xiang*)
Myrrha (*Mo Yao*)
Feces Trogopterori Seu Pteromi (*Wu Ling Zhi*)
Cinnabar (*Zhu Sha*)

The use of either of these two formulas is meant to transform stasis, regulate the menstruation, and stop pain. *Nei Yi II Fang* is for use if there is both lower abdominal pain with incessant bleeding due to vacuity cold of the *chong* and *ren*.

4. Ma Min-zhen's Protocol[4]

In this protocol, 83 cases of endometriosis were treated with *Xue Fu Zhu Yu Tang* based on the assumption that endometriosis always involves blood stasis. Ma identifies endometriosis with the TCM disease category of *zheng jia*, concretion and conglomeration. According to Ma, endometriosis is basically an accumulation and gathering (*ji ju*) disease condition within the abdomen due mostly to cold congelation, qi stagnation, and qi and blood insufficiency. These various mechanisms cause stasis and accumulation within the blood vessels and stagnation and retention in the channels and connecting vessels. Block and blockage of the tunnels (*sui dao*) result in lack of patency or free flow in transportation and movement of the qi and blood of the *chong* and *ren*. Blood is thus forced outside its channels and is retained outside its vessels. This results in stasis and binding in the lower burner with binding turning into concretion.

Based on these assumptions, Ma prescribed *Xue Fu Zhu Yu Tang* as the main or guiding formula in this research protocol. Ma then modified this formula depending upon the individual pattern discrimination and according to the principles of warming the *jing* (channels/menses) and scattering cold; soothing the liver and rectifying the qi; clearing heat and transforming dampness; boosting and moving the qi; and quickening the blood and transforming stasis. If endometriosis is complicated by infertility, Ma says that one should also supplement the kidneys along with medicinals designed to accomplish these other ends. This is based on the fact that, in TCM, the root of reproduction is not separable from the kidneys.

However, in addition to the internally administered medicinals, Ma also prescribed a retention enema. I have mentioned above in the

---

[4]   Ma Min-zhen, "The Treatment of 83 Cases of Endometriosis with *Xue Fu Zhu Yu Tang*," *Shang Hai Zhong Yi Yao Za Zhi (Shanghai Journal of TCM)*, No. 2, 1993, p.16-17

chapter on fallopian tube blockage that various modern Chinese protocols for that condition have begun to use retention enemas and that I thought that approach might also be profitably used in the treatment of endometriosis. This research corroborates and validates that opinion.

Rx: *Xue Fu Zhu Yu Tang*

Radix Angelicae Sinensis (*Dang Gui*)
Radix Rehmanniae (*Sheng Di*)
Flos Carthami Tinctorii (*Hong Hua*)
Radix Rubrus Paeoniae Lactiflorae (*Chi Shao*)
Radix Achyranthis Bidentatae (*Niu Xi*)
Fructus Citri Seu Ponciri (*Zhi Ke*)
Radix Platycodi Grandiflori (*Jie Geng*)
Rhizoma Ligustici Wallichii (*Chuan Xiong*)
Radix Glycyrrhizae (*Gan Cao*)
Radix Bupleuri (*Chai Hu*)
Semen Pruni Persicae (*Tao Ren*)

Additions & subtractions based on pattern discrimination: For cold congelation and blood stasis, in order to warm the *jing* (channels/menses) and scatter cold, add Herba Cum Radice Asari Seiboldi (*Xi Xin*) and Radix Praeparatus Aconiti Carmichaeli (*Fu Zi*). For qi stagnation and blood stasis, in order to soothe the liver and rectify the qi, add Fructus Meliae Toosendanis (*Chuan Lian Zi*), Pollen Typhae (*Pu Huang*), and Feces Trogopterori Seu Pteromi (*Wu Ling Zhi*). For heat depression and blood stasis, in order to clear heat and transform dampness, add Caulis Sargentodoxae (*Hong Teng*) and Herba Patriniae Heterophyllae (*Bai Jiang Cao*). For qi vacuity and blood stasis, in order to boost and move the qi, add Radix Astragali Membranacei (*Huang Qi*), Radix Codonopsis Pilosulae (*Dang Shen*), and Radix Saussureae Seu Vladimiriae (*Mu Xiang*). For lumps within the pelvis, add Rhizoma Sparganii (*San Leng*) and Rhizoma Curcumae Zedoariae (*E Zhu*). For infertility, in order to supplement the kidneys, quicken the blood, and transform stasis, add Herba Epimedii (*Xian*

Ling Pi), Rhizoma Curculiginis Orchoidis (*Xian Mao*), and Semen Cuscutae (*Tu Si Zi*).

Retention Enema:

Rhizoma Sparganii (*San Leng*)
Rhizoma Curcumae Zedoariae (*E Zhu*)
Caulis Sargentodoxae (*Hong Teng*)
Spina Gleditschiae Chinensis (*Jiao Zao Ci*)
Nidus Vespae (*Feng Fang*)
Radix Rubrus Paeoniae Lactiflorae (*Chi Shao*)
Semen Pruni Persicae (*Tao Ren*)

Decoct the above down to 50 ml of liquid and administer as an enema. Retain for 15 minutes; 1 treatment per day.

According to Ma, all 83 cases treated with the above protocol showed signs and symptoms of blood stasis. The ages of the women in this study ranged from 21-53 years old, with the average being 36. The shortest disease duration among this group was 1 year and the longest was 12 years. Twenty-six women suffered from concomitant infertility. Thirty-six had histories of artificial abortion. Sixty-four had dysmenorrhea. Twenty-six had dyspareunia or pain with intercourse. Fifty-four had menstrual irregularity. Twenty-eight had pelvic adhesions. And 8 had enlarged uteri.

Of the 83 cases treated as above, 41 were cured and 23 conceived. Another 27 experienced marked improvement and 10, fair improvement. Five women experienced no result. Thus, the total amelioration rate as typically figured in Chinese TCM journal articles was 94%.

5. Zhu & Cheng's Protocol[5]

This protocol is based on the use of blood-quickening, stasis-transforming medicinals on 53 women with endometriosis. The authors, Zhu Wen-xin and Cheng Xiao-an, say that this approach is based on clinical experience contained in the *Ji Yin Gang Mu (Detailed Outline for Aiding Yin [i.e., Women])* and on the fact that endometriosis is categorized in TCM as blood stasis in the lower abdomen. The 53 women in the treatment group presented with menstrual pain, menstrual irregularity, ovarian cysts, and enlarged uteri. These women were compared with 10 women with normal menstruation who served as a control group. Treatment consisted of internally administered medicinals given in decoction combined with retention enemas.

Rx:

1. Orally administered medicinals included (more or less)

Radix Salviae Miltiorrhizae (*Dan Shen*)
Cortex Radicis Moutan (*Dan Pi*)
Radix Rubrus Paeoniae Lactiflorae (*Chi Shao*)
Pollen Typhae (*Pu Huang*)
Feces Trogopterori Seu Pteromi (*Wu Ling Zhi*)
Rhizoma Corydalis Yanhusuo (*Yan Hu*)
Semen Pruni Persicae (*Tao Ren*)
Hirudo (*Shui Zhi*)
Spica Prunellae Vulgaris (*Xia Gu Cao*)
Caulis Sargentodoxae (*Hong Teng*), etc.

---

[5] Zhu Wen-xin & Cheng Xiao-an, "Clinical Study on the Treatment of Endometriosis with Blood-activating, Stasis-transforming Method," *Zhong Guo Zhong Xi Yi Jie He Za Zhi (Journal of Integrated Chinese-Western Medicine)*, No. 1, 1993, p. 16-17

2. Retention enema medicinals included (more or less)

Herba Oldenlandiae Diffusae (*Bai Hua She She Cao*)
Herba Patriniae Heterophyllae (*Bai Jiang Cao*)
Radix Arnebiae Seu Lithospermi (*Zi Cao Gen*)
Radix Salviae Miltiorrhizae (*Dan Shen*)
Cortex Phellodendri (*Huang Bai*), etc.

The average length of treatment was 3.5 months, with the average number of *ji* for internal decoctions being 105 (88-108) and for retention enemas 102 (84-168). Women were analyzed using the hemodynamic index of uterine arterial blood flow. After treatment, the uterine arteries of the 53 women significantly decreased and uterine blood flow speed reduced markedly from before treatment. These indices in the treatment group had been significantly higher before treatment than the normal, control group. After treatment, dysmenorrhea and menstrual irregularity disappeared. Twenty-two ovarian cysts became smaller and 16 disappeared. The pregnancy rate was 45%. According to the authors of this study, the data collected suggests that the Western biological mechanisms associated with TCM methods of quickening the blood and transforming stasis may be closely related to regulation of the physicochemical characteristics of the blood and the adjustment of the function of hemodynamics.

9

Female Immunologic Infertility

In Chinese, *nu xing mian gan xing bu yun zheng* or female immunologic infertility refers to various allergic reactions some women have to male sperm. These women produce antibodies which either immobilize, agglutinate, or kill their sexual partner's sperm and thus render fertilization impossible. Such immunologic infertility may account for approximately 20% of infertility. Hou Ling-ling, in a recent article whose English title translates as "A Preliminary Exploration of Female Immunologic Infertility," remarks that this disease category is obviously not a TCM one.[1] So far, no recognized TCM differentiation of patterns for this disease category has been established. In some cases, this condition goes along with inflammation of the uterus and fallopian tubes due to external invasion or undisciplined sexual behavior. However, this cannot be said about all women with this condition.

Although I will have more to say about this condition under candidiasis below, Hou suggests that the treatment principles for correcting this condition can be discussed under five headings.

1. Quickening the blood

First of all, Hou says that the primary therapy should be to quicken the blood. This is in part based on the Western scientific fact that the

---

[1]   Hou Ling-ling, "A Preliminary Exploration of Female Immunologic Fertility," *Zhong Yi Za Zhi (Journal of TCM)*, Vol. 33, No. 5, p. 14-15

actions of many if not most *huo xue* medicinals can also be classified as anti-inflammatory. In addition, they regulate the *chong* and *ren* and seem to also regulate immunity. The medicinals Huo uses as examples are:

Radix Pseudoginseng (*San Qi*)
Radix Salviae Miltiorrhizae (*Dan Shen*)
Radix Angelicae Sinensis (*Dang Gui*)
Semen Pruni Persicae (*Tao Ren*)
Flos Carthami Tinctorii (*Hong Hua*)
Flos Seu Herba Schizonepetae Tenuifoliae (*Jing Jie*)
Herba Leonuri Heterophylli (*Yi Mu Cao*)

2. Clearing & resolving stasis & toxins

The second group of medicinals Hou suggests using are those which are anti-inflammatory and antimicrobial but which are not too bitter and cold and which also quicken the blood, scatter nodulation, and regulate immunity, such as:

Herba Andrographidis (*Chuan Xin Lian*)
Spica Prunellae Vulgaris (*Xia Gu Cao*)
Herba Houttuyniae Cordatae (*Yu Xing Cao*)
Radix Sophorae Flavescentis (*Ku Shen*) etc.

3. Purging, disinhibiting, sweeping away, & scattering

The examples of medicinals fulfilling these principles given by Hou include:

Radix Et Rhizoma Rhei (*Da Huang*)
Sclerotium Poriae Cocoris (*Fu Ling*)
Rhizoma Alismatis (*Ze Xie*)
Radix Bupleuri (*Chai Hu*)
Ramulus Cinnamomi (*Gui Zhi*) etc.

Radix Et Rhizoma Rhei precipitates heat, sweeps away evils, quickens the blood, and is antimicrobial. Sclerotium Poriae Cocoris and Rhizoma Alismatis disinhibit urination. Radix Bupleuri courses, sweeps away, and disinhibits urination at the same time as it is anti-inflammatory. Ramulus Cinnamomi warms and scatters while it quickens the blood. These medicinals can waste yin, however, and so they should be combined with yin-supplementing, yin-enriching medicinals, such as:

Radix Glehniae Littoralis (*Sha Shen*)
Tuber Ophiopogonis Japonicae (*Mai Dong*)
Rhizoma Anemarrhenae (*Zhi Mu*)

4. Boosting the *chong* & *ren*

From a modern TCM point of view, supplementing and boosting the *chong* and *ren* are necessary to promote conception. If there are antisperm antibodies, Hou says it is also very important to supplement and boost the *chong* and *ren*, nourish the blood and consolidate the fetus since there is the danger of likely miscarriage. The medicinals Hou suggests from this category are:

Semen Cuscutae (*Tu Si Zi*)
Radix Dipsaci (*Chuan Duan*)
Cortex Eucommiae Ulmoidis (*Du Zhong*)
prepared Radix Rehmanniae (*Shu Di*)
Fructus Lycii Chinensis (*Gou Qi Zi*)
Fructus Ligustri Lucidi (*Nu Zhen Zi*) etc.

5. Conjointly treating the man

For the treatment of agglutinated sperm, the reader is referred to *A Handbook of Traditional Chinese Urology & Male Sexual Dysfunction* by Anna Lin, also published by Blue Poppy Press.

Hou gives three case histories in his article, none of which are particularly remarkable or revealing. In each case, the patient's TCM pattern was ascertained via the four diagnoses and a formula was written which would also regulate and cure any menstrual irregularity. However, in one case, vaginal washes were used. In this case, the woman was diagnosed as suffering from yang vacuity of the *chong* and *ren* with liver depression and blood stagnation. A formula, not given in the article, was administered orally in order to warm the *chong* and *ren*, course the liver, and quicken the blood. A liquid extract of Flos Carthami Tinctorii (*Hong Hua*) was used to irrigate the vagina and cervix. Once the patient's lower abdominal period pain was eliminated, this was supplanted by washing the vagina and cervix with an injectable extract of Radix Salviae Miltiorrhizae (*Dan Shen*).

As mentioned above, I will have more to say about female immunologic infertility and sperm allergies below. However, the use of a wash or douche to the vagina and cervix directly with Chinese medicinals is a logical addition to the oral treatment of this condition and is an approach which merits much further consideration and research. If an infection is found in the reproductive tract, Chinese medicinals can be chosen with a known antimicrobial effect on those pathogens. Too often, Western physicians fail to identify the real culprit microbe provoking a hyperimmune or allergic response. In my experience in such cases, it is wise to use antimycotic medicinals.

1. Chen Xiao-ping *et al.*'s Protocol[2]

Chen Xiao-ping, Chen Dan-ping, and Dong Gui-hong describe their treatment of 85 women with immunologic infertility in the December, 1992 issue of the *Zhong Yi Za Zhi (The Journal of Traditional Chinese Medicine)*. Of the 85 women studied, 31 were from 25-30

---

[2] Chen Xiao-ping, Chen Dan-ping, & Dong Gui-hong, "The Treatment of Immunologic Infertility with *Gu Yin Jian* and its Effect on Humoral Immunity," *Zhong Yi Za Zhi (Journal of TCM)*, No. 12, 1992, p. 36-37

210

years old; 49 were from 31-40; and 5 were 41 or older. Sixty women were treated with internally administered Chinese herbal decoctions. The remaining 25 were used as a comparative control group. These women were given 100 mg of vitamin E and 5 mg of Prednisone per day. The TCM formula used was based on the assumption that supplementing the kidneys is a main therapeutic principle in the treatment of infertility.

Rx: *Gu Yin Jian*

Radix Panacis Ginseng (*Sheng Shai Shen*)
prepared Radix Rehmanniae (*Da Shu Di*)
Radix Dioscoreae Oppositae (*Shan Yao*)
Fructus Corni Officinalis (*Shan Zhu Rou*)
Semen Cuscutae (*Tu Si Zi*)
processed Radix Polygalae Tenuifoliae (*Yuan Zhi*)
Fructus Schizandrae Chinensis (*Wu Wei Zi*)
mix-fried Radix Glycyrrhizae (*Zhi Gan Cao*)

Thirty days of treatment was considered one course of therapy and treatment was discontinued if no result was obtained after 3 full courses. Treatment efficacy was measured by monthly semen immune tests (SIT). In the group treated with Chinese herbal medicine, 19 women were cured or 37.7%, 32 women improved (53.3%), and 9 women or 15% experienced no result. In the control group which received modern Western medicine, 6 women (24%) were cured, 8 improved (32%), and 11 (44%) experienced no result.

Although this study suggests that traditional Chinese medicine is more effective than modern Western medicine for the treatment of this condition, analysis of changes in serum or humoral immune factors is also enlightening. Serum levels of IgA, IgG, and IgM were measured before and after treatment. In the group treated with Chinese herbal medicine, IgA levels decreased significantly, IgG levels went up significantly, and IgM levels stayed statistically about the same. Among the women treated with modern Western medicine, there were no statistically significant changes in serum levels of any of these three immunoglobulins.

IgA is found in seromucous secretions of the body tracts exposed to the external environment, such as saliva, tears, and presumably vaginal secretions. It provides an early antibacterial and antiviral defense. Post-treatment reductions in IgA suggest that the women's vagina secretions might be less hostile to foreign microbes, including male sperm. IgG, on the other hand, is the most prevalent type of serum Ig. It is a prime mediator in the secondary immune response. IgG can also inhibit some antigen-antibody reactions and one suggested mechanism for desensitization in atopic allergies is the development of blocking IgG antibodies which prevent IgE antigen reactions. IgE is elevated in atopic diseases, such as allergic asthma, atopic dermatitis, and possibly female allergies to sperm. In addition, according to Chen *et al.*, these medicinals are able to regulate and adjust hypothalamus, pituitary, ovarian, and uterine hormonal secretions, thus promoting conception.

212

10

Candidiasis & Infertility

Over the last several years, I have become increasingly convinced that the large intestine plays a greater role in the health of human beings than that for which modern TCM credits it. In particular, I have observed that dysbiosis of the bowels is typically present in many complicated, chronic, and recalcitrant conditions. In *Scatology & the Gate of Life*, I have preliminarily discussed the connections between the large intestine and the kidneys and their role in immunity.[1] In addition, in that book I have discussed the possibility and ramifications of diagnosing candidiasis as a species of intestinal parasite or *chong* according to TCM logic. Since 1990 when I wrote that book, I have become more and not less convinced that candidiasis is an important factor in the TCM diagnosis and treatment of a host of disorders and not least of all female endocrinopathies.

In William G. Crook's *The Yeast Connection*, Dr. Crook describes the connection between candidiasis, PMS, endometriosis, and infertility.[2] His opinions are based on and corroborated by the clinical experience of Drs. C. Orrian Truss, Richard Mabray, and A. Stephen Orr, the later two being gynecologists. John Parks Trow-

---

[1]   Flaws, Bob, *Scatology and the Gate of Life: The Role of the Large Intestine in Immunity, An Integrated Chinese-Western Approach*, Blue Poppy Press, Boulder, CO, 1990

[2]   Crook, William G., *The Yeast Connection*, Vintage Books, Random House, New York, 1986

bridge, MD, also sees vaginitis, vulval itching, cystitis, menstrual disorders, premenstrual syndrome, sexual difficulties, decreased libido, and infertility among a host of other diseases and pathological conditions as all possibly related to candidiasis. As a TCM doctor specializing in *fu ke* or gynecology, it is certainly my experience that polysystemic chronic candidiasis (PSCC) can and typically does play a large part in the above gynecological disorders amongst American patients.

Candida albicans is a commensal, saprophytic yeast. Commensal means that it normally inhabits our body, *i.e.*, it lives with us in the house of our body. It is a part of our normal, internal ecology. Saprophyte means that its role in the body is to scavenge and eat debris similar to yeasts and fungi which break down garbage in a compost heap. These commensal yeast have their proper home in our intestines. Their populations and activities are held in check by both our host immune system and the other commensal protozoa (*fauna*) and bacteria (*flora*) of the intestinal tract with which they have synergistic relationships. Normally the walls of the large intestine are sufficiently impermeable so that these yeast remain within the confines of the bowels. However, if the intestinal lining becomes more permeable, yeast bodies can migrate outside the intestines. They may also migrate up the alimentary tract and thence outward into the body.

Yeast move outward from the intestines by sending out hyphae or tentacles between the body's cell walls. These then bud and release spores resulting in new yeast bodies. Within the bowels themselves, whose hollows it should be remembered are an extension of the outside of the body, mostly it is the good intestinal bacteria which keep *Candida* populations in check. However, once these yeast travel outside the large intestine's confines and enter the inside of the body itself, it is the job of the immune system to neutralize and remove these foreign invaders. Therefore, there are three elements to keep in mind when considering the body's ability to maintain a proper homeostatic, symbiotic relationship with *Candida albicans*: 1) the

intestinal ecology of yeasts, bacteria, and protozoa; 2) the imperme-
ability of the intestinal lining; and 3) the competence of the host
immune system.

The immune system is comprised of two distinct classes of cells
whose job it is to identify and neutralize foreign proteins and invading
microbes, whether they be protozoa, bacteria, or yeast and fungi.
However, it is the endocrine system which regulates much of the
activity of the immune system through the release of various
hormones and steroids. In a sense, the endocrine system gives the
immune system many of its marching orders, and thus the competence
of the immune system is somewhat dependent on a properly functioning endocrine system.

Yeast within the body protect themselves from predation by the host
immune system by manufacturing and secreting hormone analogues
to foil the immune system. As Dr. Trowbridge puts it:

> All of us yeast build molecules disguised to look similar to
> hormonal molecules. Some of these disguises become our surface
> antigens; they allow us to enter our universes's cellular communi-
> cation traffic. I slip into Jane's metabolic process of cell communi-
> cation and give her sleepless nights, cramp-filled days, and painful
> sexual intercourse.[3]

In other words, these hormone-like substances give the body's
immune cells the wrong marching orders. However, in the process
and because the endocrine system functions via a feedback loop, these
wrong signals to the endocrine glands upset the delicate balance of the
endocrine system's regulation of many other of the body's metabolic
functions. In women, these wrong signals can wreak havoc with
ovulation, gestation, and menstruation. Thus we begin to see how

---

[3]   Trowbridge, John Parks & Walker, Morton, *The Yeast Syndrome*, Bantam
       Books, Toronto, 1988, p. 18

candidiasis, the pathological proliferation of *Candida albicans* within the body, can cause or at least participate in all sorts of menstrual and reproductive disorders, including endometriosis and infertility.

Unfortunately, that is not the entire story. When yeast invade the body from the intestines, they proliferate and die. When they die, they break down into their chemical components. These breakdown products include yeast proteins which the body recognizes as foreign. The body's response to foreign proteins within the body is to mount an immune response. This includes the release of histamine. If the body is constantly provoked into such immune responses, we can talk of an allergic response. This is a histamine response to something which, under normal circumstances in an healthy individual should not cause a histamine reaction. Such allergies are a hyperimmune response. If this continues over and over again, over time this hyperimmune reaction can result in two things: 1) The immune system may go into overdrive and become autoimmune. This means that it starts creating antibodies to its own proteins in a fit of endocrine neurotic paranoia; and 2) the immune system becomes exhausted and, therefore, less able to adequately deal with all sorts of pathogens it would ordinarily be expected to neutralize.

Many women with PSCC suffer from autoimmune ovaritis and thyroiditis. This means inflammation and resulting dysfunction of these glands due to, in the case of the ovaries, antiovarian antibodies. It is well known in modern Western medicine that many women who complain of infertility have hypothyroid function and that thyroid function enhancing therapies can result in restoring fertility. It is also well known that luteal phase progesterone deficiency may also cause infertility and is due to hypofunction of the ovaries. As we have seen above, both these conditions can be due to an autoimmune response triggered by PSCC. In addition, PSCC may also result in a woman's creating antisperm antibodies which attack and kill either a particular man's or all men's sperm. This may also cause female infertility.

In the case of luteal phase defect, the situation seems to be even more convoluted. Progesterone is well known to aggravate candidiasis. At midcycle, the corpus luteum begins secreting progesterone. This causes an increase in *Candida* populations in the body. On the one hand, these *Candida* populations secrete an estrogen-like analogue which causes symptoms of PMS, such as swollen, tender breasts, due to seeming hyperestrogenosis. On the other hand, as they naturally die and their endotoxins are liberated into the system, this provokes an allergic reaction. If the body's immune system is already dysfunctional and autoimmune, this allergic die-off reaction may cause autoimmune ovaritis. This then impedes the ovaries' continued production of progesterone and leads to a shortened menstrual cycle due to progesterone deficiency. Then, when the progesterone levels drop dramatically, there is a massive yeast die-off and all hell breaks loose in the woman's body—nausea, vomiting, chills, flu-like aches and pains, abdominal cramping, diarrhea, etc.

Phyllis Saifer, MD, has coined the term autoimmune polyendrocrino-pathy immune-dysregulation candidiasis hypersensitivity syndrome or APICH syndrome for short. This syndrome can help explain the broad reaching, systemic effects the seemingly innocuous yeast, *Candida albicans*, can have on human health and disease as outlined above. Unfortunately, women are more at risk for PSCC and APICH than men. This is because their monthly cycle and pregnancy involve hormonal shifts which cause fluctuations of immune competence and can, therefore, allow proliferation of *Candida* outside the intestines. Secondly, women are much more prone to the types of infections, in part provoked by candidiasis, for which modern Western physicians routinely prescribe antibiotics, such as cystitis, vaginitis, and PID. These antibiotics often kill off the healthy intestinal flora which keep *Candida* populations in check. Once this biological control mechanism is absent, yeast populations may swell and begin migrating outside the intestines. And third, hormone therapies, such as oral birth control pills, estrogen-replacement therapy, and various corticosteroids may all tip the balance of internal humoral balance, thus decreasing immune competence and allowing yeast to multiply and invade.

Even more unfortunately, the modern American diet only exacerbates PSCC. Monosaccharides are like jet fuel to yeast. Therefore, a diet high in carbohydrates and sweets feeds yeast populations. This includes glucose, lactose, and fructose or, we could say, grain products, milk products, and fruits. Further, the sweeter a food or drink is, the more likely it is to provoke a yeast overgrowth. In addition, any foods contaminated with large numbers of yeast bodies will tend to provoke an allergic reaction in persons with PSCC. When a person eats cheese or drinks alcohol or eats anything made with vinegar, these foods are not adding live, viable yeast to the patient's already overburdened body. But they do add dead yeast bodies which means yeast proteins. These proteins are absorbed through the gastrointestinal lining and provoke an allergic reaction in the body whose immune system has been irritated and aggravated by chronic candidiasis. In some people, their intestinal lining becomes so permeable that other large proteins from foods are also able to get into the blood stream and provoke allergic responses. These people typically speak about their multiple food allergies, for instance to wheat, corn, eggs, and dairy. If such a hyperimmune/allergic condition is really severe, patients can be made sick by simply inhaling foreign molecules, such as from perfume, petrochemical products, and other organic compounds.

The following is a list of *Candida* related endocrinopathies as enumerated by Dr. Saifer:[4]

1. Hypothyroidism
2. Thyroiditis
3. Hypoadrenalism
4. Diabetes mellitus

5. Hypoparathyroidism
6. Pernicious anemia
7. Hepatitis due to viral infection

---

4   *Ibid.*, p. 326-329

8. Alopecia or hair loss
9. Vitiligo
10. PMS
11. Addison's disease
12. Ovaritis
13. Myasthenia gravis
14. Pemphigus
15. Allergic rhinitis
16. Schizophrenia
17. Autism
18. Sprue
19. Celiac disease
20. Idiopathic thrombocytopenic purpura
21. Testiculitis
22. Pituitary deficiency with amenorrhea
23. Systemic lupus erythmatosis
24. Rheumatoid arthritis
25. Sjogren's syndrome
26. Goodpasture's syndrome

Dr. Saifer is quoted by Dr. Trowbridge as saying, "All of the above twenty-six conditions of APICH syndrome are autoimmune diseases in which antibodies to 'self' can be demonstrated."[5] Dr. Trowbridge goes on to say, "They are systemic autoimmune problems, and a distinct relationship to the Candida syndrome appears likely."[6] Certainly that is my clinical experience.

From a TCM Perspective

All the above is basically a modern Western medical description of the effects of candidiasis on the immune and endocrine systems. Without doubt, some modern Western doctors, such as Trowbridge, Truss, Mabray, Orr, Saifer, and Crook, see a relationship between PSCC and endometriosis and infertility. But what does this mean in TCM terms?

As mentioned above, *Candida albicans* can be described in TCM terms as a *chong* or parasite. It is so described in modern Chinese *fu ke* texts when discussing vaginitis. In those same discussions, modern

---

[5]   *Ibid.*, p. 329

[6]   *Ibid.*, p.329

Chinese gynecologists, such as Han Bai-ling, say that these yeasts' normal home is within the stomach and intestines. According to TCM, *chong* tend to arise in a damp hot environment or are associated with evil dampness and heat. Often this damp heat is also associated with spleen vacuity. The spleen controls the transportation and transformation of body fluids. If the spleen becomes weak and deficient, either through excessive thinking, overtaxation, or faulty diet, it may fail to *yun* and *hua* liquids and body fluids. These, being heavy, may then percolate downward to the lower burner. If dampness collects, it can obstruct the free flow of qi and blood in the lower burner. In addition, by obstructing the qi, the qi may back up and transform into heat, thus giving rise to dampness and heat. This provides the perfect environment for the arisal of *chong* according to TCM.

However, things are not as simple as that. Every case of PSCC is not simply one of damp heat in the lower burner or even damp heat mixed by spleen vacuity. Qi stagnation may lead to blood stasis and this may adversely injure and damage the kidneys. The kidneys typically are also damaged by both dampness and heat. Dampness, being yin, injures kidney qi which is yang. Likewise, evil heat also wastes and injures righteous qi. Therefore, it is not uncommon to see kidney yang vacuity below as well. At first this looks contradictory, but in clinical practice it is not. As we will see below, there are a number of formulas in TCM which are designed to treat just this scenario.

Further, yang being vacuous below, it loses its root or lower source and tends to flush up. Since heat injures and damages true water or righteous body fluids, this often causes signs and symptoms of heat and dryness or yin vacuity above. And, as if that were not enough, heat and dampness obstructing and hindering the free and patent flow of qi and blood in the lower burner directly impinge upon the liver's function of ruling, coursing, and discharge and especially in the lower burner. This then tends to aggravate any preexisting liver depression and qi stagnation and may even give rise to depressive fire. Therefore, it is entirely possible to see patients with a combination of dampness and heat below, yang vacuity and cold below, qi and blood stasis, and spleen and yin vacuity.

In my experience as a TCM gynecologist practicing in the United States, this complicated scenario is also a relatively common one. If one understands polysystemic chronic candidiasis and APICH syndrome, it can help to make all the above elements more understandable. Likewise, it can help improve one's prescription writing, help design appropriate and indispensably important dietary modifications, and help explain seemingly adverse or unexpected reactions to TCM formulas or medicinals.

PSCC & the Four Diagnoses

Candidiasis as a species of *chong* is a disease diagnosis. It is not a pattern or *zheng* as such. In modern TCM, disease diagnoses may be made by means other than the traditional *si zhen* or four diagnoses. Nowadays, disease diagnoses may be made on the basis of laboratory findings. However, even using the four diagnoses alone, the TCM practitioner can make a pretty accurate diagnosis of PSCC.

Questioning

As in modern TCM in general, the most important method is questioning. In particular, the practitioner is interested if the patient has or has had any of the following conditions: PMS, vaginitis, cystitis, constipation, diarrhea, flatulence, bloating, belching, indigestion, heartburn, food allergies or intolerances, sinusitis, canker sores or blisters in the mouth, fungal skin infections, hives, eczema, psoriasis, and acne, lump in throat, falling hair, or dandruff. Are any of these conditions aggravated by eating sweets, carbohydrates, yeasted, or fermented foods? Are any of these conditions aggravated cyclically along with one's menstrual cycle? Has one had a recent or prolonged courses of antibiotic therapy? Has or is one using any type of hormone therapy, including the Pill? Are any of the patient's

221

symptoms aggravated by damp weather or exposure to mold? Affirmative answers to questions such as these suggest possible candidiasis.

Inspection

In terms of inspection, the tongue can often help confirm candidiasis. Of course, if the patient has oral thrush, that is pretty conclusive, but it is also not commonly encountered by the gynecologist. If the tongue has a yellow, dryish or greasy coating with bald patches or the tongue is red and cracked with a geographic coating and hurts if the patient eats tomatoes or oranges, this is pretty conclusive of candidiasis in my experience. Canker sores and tongue sores are also indicative. A thick, slimy yellow coating at the base of the tongue, suggests damp heat in the lower burner. If other signs and symptoms suggest candidiasis, this then can be seen as an indication of it as well. However, people with candidiasis may have a relatively normal tongue coating. A fluted tongue and inner cheeks marked with the indentations of the teeth suggest at the very least that the spleen is not transporting and transforming liquids properly and is a strong indication of dampness.

Modern TCM textbooks on tongue diagnosis, such as Giovanni Maciocia's *Tongue Diagnosis in Chinese Medicine*,[7] most commonly say that cracks on the lingual surface indicate injury and damage of yin fluids. However, Sun Bin-yan, a renowned Chinese cancer specialist whose work is strongly influenced by Li Dong-yuan, says that such cracks indicate vacuity of original qi.[8] This original qi refers to the middle qi which is the origin of all postnatally produced

---

[7] Maciocia, Giovanni, *Tongue Diagnosis in Chinese Medicine*, Eastland Press, Seattle, WA, 1987

[8] Sun, Bin-yan, *Cancer Treatment and Prevention with Traditional Chinese Medicine*, Effete Enterprises Inc., San Mateo, CA, 1991, p.53

222

qi and blood. This underscores the fact that when there is candidiasis, often there is dryness and vacuity of stomach fluids and lung and heart yin coexisting with a damp, deficient spleen. If heat associated with damp heat has wafted up and injured fluids above, not only will there be cracks, but the tongue may be red as well or at least its tip. Even so, such cracks should also be read as indicating a spleen qi vacuity which is so often at the root of the damp hot environment conducive to the flourishing of *chong*.

Some Chinese doctors read a central vertical crack as indicating a vacuity problem of the heart. Others feel that this indicates a *chong mai* problem. And yet others suggest that such a vertical crack indicates a vacuity problem in the viscera associated with the region of the tongue the crack traverses. Therefore, a crack near the tip indicates a vacuity problem of the heart; a crack in the central portion indicates a vacuity of the spleen; and a crack in the rear indicates a vacuity of the kidneys. Since the *chong mai* connects the heart with the kidneys and regulates the liver and the spleen and stomach, these various points of view are not mutually contradictory or exclusive.

According to Li Dong-yuan, damp heat in the lower burner can enter the blood *fen* and the *chong mai* is the sea of blood. The heat component can rise up along the *chong mai* to the heart. Heat accumulating in the heart disturbs the *shen*. Heat accumulating in the lungs can impede the lungs' diffusion of qi and body fluids. Heat rising up the *chong mai* can also affect the liver and spleen's relationship, throwing them out of balance. All this is discussed in Li Dong-yuan's *Pi Wei Lun (Treatise of the Spleen & Stomach)* when he talks about the systemic effects of yin fire.[9]

Li's yin fire is none other than damp heat. Dampness is yin and fire is heat. As we have seen above, it is damp heat that provides the

---

[9]   Li Dong-yuan, *Treatise on the Spleen and Stomach*, translated by Yang Shou-zhong and Li Jian-yong, Blue Poppy Press, Boulder, CO, 1993

terrain in which *chong*, such as *Candida albicans*, flourish. There-fore, a vertical crack in the center of the tongue typically suggests a problem with the *chong mai* and such problems are commonly associated with yin fire and candidiasis. Thus this sign is also suggestive of this condition.

Palpation

As for the pulse, most often I look at the *chi* or foot positions for confirmation of candidiasis. If the right *chi* is somewhat deep but then slippery, this suggests both damp heat in the lower burner and surging upwards of *ming men* fire. If *yuan qi* is vacuous below, it may fail to hold liver/kidney fire in place. These two mechanisms are not unrelated. If the left *chi* is soggy or *ru mai*, this suggests kidney yin vacuity with vacuity cold in the lower burner. The soggy pulse is defined as a pulse which feels floating, very thready, and without strength. It is like a strand of cotton floating on water and feels very thin and indistinct. It is like a bubble which bursts when pressure is lightly increased. The soft pulse usually indicates damage to the *ying* and blood and severe vacuity of yin *jing*. It can also indicate spleen vacuity with inability to control dampness.

The Fingernail Lunulae

Often there seems to be a confusing mixture of hot and cold, vacuity and repletion, dryness and dampness. It should be remembered that the tongue is in the upper part of the body. Although it is believed to reflect the entire body, still heat, because it tends to float upwards, reflects strongly in the tongue as does dryness and yin vacuity above caused by such heat. Whereas, cold feet, cold extremities, long, frequent, clear urination, fear of cold, and the lunulae of fingernails often bespeak of simultaneous cold and dampness. Sun Bin-yan, mentioned above, believes that the lunulae, the little crescents at the base of the fingernails, indicate the presence of righteous warmth in the body. If these lunulae are smaller than usual or are missing on some of the fingers, this indicates an element of vacuity cold. The more lunulae missing or too small, the more cold is a factor in the patient's condition.[10] I have found this system to be of use in clinical practice where there are both cold and hot symptoms appearing together.

Therapeutic Principles

When candidiasis plays a part in a patient's condition, this suggests using *sha chong* (killing parasites) and *qu chong* (dispelling parasites) therapy. Modern researchers in China have identified a number of medicinals which have strong antimycotic, antifungal properties and which are effective for reducing overgrowth in *Candida* populations. These include:

Rhizoma Coptidis Chinensis (*Huang Lian*)
Radix Scutellariae Baicalensis (*Huang Qin*)
Cortex Phellodendri (*Huang Bai*)
Radix Et Rhizoma Rhei (*Da Huang*)
Radix Sophorae Flavescentis (*Ku Shen*)
Radix Dictamni (*Bai Xian Pi*)
Rhizoma Belamcandae (*She Gan*)
Radix Pulsatillae Chinensis (*Bai Tou Weng*)
Radix Platycodi Grandiflori (*Jie Geng*)
Herba Houttuyniae Cordatae (*Yu Xing Cao*)
Rhizoma Polygonati (*Huang Jing*)
Radix Sophorae Subprostratae (*Shan Dou Geng*)
Cortex Pseudolaricis (*Tu Jin Pi*)
Semen Cnidii Monnieri (*She Chuang Zi*)

Most of these medicinals are bitter and cold according to TCM. However, because most people with PSCC have a mixture of vacuity

---

[10]   Sun, *op. cit.*, p. 19-33

and repletion, hot and cold, sole reliance on such bitter, cold medicinals will not solve this problem. Rather, it is necessary to use a much more modulated approach. Bitter, cold medicinals clear heat and eliminate dampness from the stomach and intestines, but they can, in excess, injure the righteous qi of the spleen and yin of the stomach. Therefore, it is usually necessary to combine such bitter, cold, antimycotic medicinals with sweet, acrid, warm medicinals which boost the qi and strengthen the spleen while aromatically permeating and transforming dampness. These include:

Radix Codonopsis Pilosulae (*Dang Shen*)
Rhizoma Pinelliae Ternatae (*Ban Xia*)
Rhizoma Atractylodis (*Cang Zhu*)
Rhizoma Atractylodis Macrocephalae (*Bai Zhu*)
Radix Dioscoreae Oppositae (*Shan Yao*)
Rhizoma Zingiberis (*Jiang*)
Fructus Amomi (*Sha Ren*)
Fructus Cardamomi (*Bai Dou Kou*)
Rhizoma Alpiniae Officinari (*Gao Liang Jiang*)
Semen Alpiniae Katsumadae (*Cao Dou Kou*)
Fructus Alpiniae Oxyphyllae (*Yi Zhi Ren*)
Semen Myristicae Fragrantis (*Rou Dou Kou*)
Fructus Piperis Longi (*Pi Ba*)
Ramulus Cinnamomi (*Gui Zhi*)
Fructus Evodiae Rutecarpae (*Wu Zhu Yu*)
Fructus Zanthoxyli Bungeani (*Chuan Jiao*)

Several of the above medicinals have been identified as having antihistaminic properties. These include: Rhizoma Zingiberis, Fructus Amomi, Fructus Cardamomi, Rhizoma Alpiniae Officinari, Semen Alpiniae Katsumadae, Rhizoma Atractylodis, and Rhizoma Atractylodis Macrocephalae. Others, such as Fructus Evodiae Rutecarpae and Fructus Zanthoxyli Bungeani, themselves are credited with antiparasitic properties.

This is interesting since, when a large number of yeast are killed through medication, this often provokes a Herxheimer reaction. This is also called a die-off reaction. If lots of yeast die in the body and begin to decompose, this floods the system with their endotoxins and foreign proteins and, in turn, results in a pronounced allergic reaction. By combining bitter, cold, antimycotics with acrid, sweet, and warm antihistaminic medicinals, the *Candida* are killed without provoking a die-off reaction.

In some cases, it is important to include purgative, precipitating medicinals to rid the body of the toxic breakdown products of dead yeast. These include:

Radix Et Rhizoma Rhei (*Da Huang*)
Mirabilitum (*Mang Xiao*)
Semen Arecae Catechu (*Bing Lang*)
Cortex Magnoliae Officinalis (*Hou Po*)

Of these precipitating ingredients, Semen Arecae Catechu is a known antiparasitic medicinal and Radix Et Rhizoma Rhei is antimycotic.

Ramulus Cinnamomi (*Gui Zhi*) deserves special mention. This medicinal is an acrid, warm surface-reliever or resolver. However, it also quickens the blood in case of blood stasis and redirects fire down to its lower source. Sun Bin-yan recommends Ramulus Cinnamomi for eliminating cold and dampness in both the middle and lower burners. Western herbalists say that Cinnamomi is a carminative and astringent and use it for flatulence and diarrhea. It is an especially important medicinal in combination with bitter, cold ingredients to dispel cold and dampness, quicken the blood and dispel stasis, and redirect the *ming men* fire back downwards. As we will see below, in the treatment of infertility, the body's righteous warmth must be maintained from ovulation to just before menstruation, and Ramulus Cinnamomi is one important medicinal to insure this.

There are also a number of other ingredients which seem to work especially well in antimycotic formulas even though they are not described in the TCM literature as having special antimycotic properties. Among the qi-rectifiers, these include Radix Saussureae Seu Vladimiriae (*Mu Xiang*), Semen Citri Reticulatae (*Ju He*), Fructus Meliae Toosendanis (*Chuan Lian Zi*), and Fructus Akebiae (*Ba Yue Zha*), the latter two having pronounced antiparasitic properties. Among the blood-rectifying medicinals, these include Radix Achyranthis Bidentatae (*Huai Niu Xi*), Radix Cyathulae (*Chuan Niu Xi*), and Rhizoma Corydalis Yanhusuo (*Yan Hu Suo*). And among the heat-clearing medicinals which also quicken the blood and dispel stasis, these include Caulis Sargentodoxae (*Hong Teng*) and Herba Patriniae Heterophyllae (*Bai Jiang Cao*).

In the treatment of *Candida*-related endocrinopathies, it is also necessary to include ingredients with known effects on the pituitary, thyroid, and ovaries. Some of these include:

Radix Angelicae Sinensis (*Dang Gui*)
Radix Glycyrrhizae (*Gan Cao*)
Rhizoma Curculiginis Orchoidis (*Xian Mao*)
Herba Epimedii (*Xian Ling Pi*)
Fructus Ligustri Lucidi (*Nu Zhen Zi*)
Semen Cuscutae (*Tu Si Zi*)
Radix Dipsaci (*Chuan Duan*)
Fructus Rubi (*Fu Pen Zi*)
Radix Dioscoreae Oppositae (*Shan Yao*)

These should be chosen based on both their Western biological research *and* their TCM descriptions and functions coordinated with a *bian zheng* diagnosis. Likewise, other medicinals may be added to a patient's formula based on a combination of disease and pattern diagnoses as appropriate.

As we have seen above in our review of some of the modern Chinese TCM journal literature devoted to female infertility, there is great emphasis on supplementing the kidneys in order to promote fertilization and maintain proper luteal phase function. Many women suffering from infertility have a defective luteal phase. They cannot maintain progesterone levels high enough or long enough and, so, even though fertilization may have taken place, the zygote cannot successfully implant and the period comes anyway. Traditionally, early periods may be due to either evil heat or qi vacuity. This evil heat may be either replete, vacuous, depressive, phlegmatic, or damp. Typically the qi vacuity is spoken of as spleen qi vacuity. However, in the modern journal literature, early periods due to progesterone insufficiency are mostly treated as kidney yang *and* spleen qi vacuities.

Since the rise in progesterone after ovulation stimulates a rise in BBT, it is logical within modern TCM to associate progesterone with kidney yang or the *ming men zhi huo*, the fire of the gate of life. Therefore, it is not uncommon to find the following medicinals being suggested to lengthen the cycle and forestall the period in patients with a luteal phase defect:

Rhizoma Curculiginis Orchoidis (*Xian Mao*)
Herba Epimedii (*Xian Ling Pi*)
Radix Morindae Officinalis (*Ba Ji Tian*)
Herba Cistanchis (*Rou Cong Rong*)
Semen Cuscutae (*Tu Si Zi*)
Radix Dipsaci (*Xu Duan*)
Cortex Eucommiae Ulmoidis (*Du Zhong*)

These are commonly combined with qi-boosting, spleen-fortifiers such as:

Radix Panacis Ginseng (*Ren Shen*)
Radix Codonopsis Pilosulae (*Dang Shen*)

229

Radix Astragali Membranacei (*Huang Qi*)
Rhizoma Atractylodis Macrocephalae (*Bai Zhu*)
Radix Bupleuri (*Chai Hu*)
Rhizoma Cimicifugae (*Sheng Ma*)

Both Li Dong-yuan historically and Sun Bin-yan contemporaneously consider the last two medicinals qi-boosters and spleen-fortifiers as opposed to merely surface-relievers. Radix Bupleuri is credited with antihistaminic properties and Rhizoma Cimicifugae is a powerful antifungal even though it is not listed as such above. One of the hallmarks of Li Dong-yuan's formulas is the use of Rhizoma Cimicifugae and Cortex Phellodendri (*Huang Bai*) with Radix Panacis Ginseng, Radix Astragali Membranacei, Rhizoma Atractylodis Macrocephalae, and Rhizoma Atractylodis (*Cang Zhu*).

In my experience, often there is an element of heat in cases of early periods with luteal phase defect. The explanation for this, I believe, is that, as described above, progesterone stimulates a yeast explosion in the body. These proliferating yeast then cause an autoimmune assault on the ovaries and possibly also the thyroid. This causes the ovaries to stop producing sufficient progesterone and even perhaps the thyroid to stop producing thyroid hormone. Thus the BBT plummets and the period arrives early. The woman is distraught and this further upsets the endocrine system through the neocortex's connection to the pituitary via the hypophysis/hypothalamus.

Therefore, in order to break this vicious cycle, some attention to controlling yeast populations is necessary while at the same time warming the kidneys and uterus and maintaining the BBT. Radix Bupleuri and Rhizoma Cimicifugae, being cold in nature, help in keeping yeast populations down. When these two acrid, bitter, and cold medicinals are combined with another acrid, bitter, cold ingredient with strong antimycotic properties, such as Cortex Phellodendri, the effect is even better. Thus once again, one is talking about a combination of acrid, warm and bitter, cold medicinals

230

employed simultaneously to kill yeast but prevent a die-off allergic reaction.

Formulas

The TCM literature includes a number of formulas which address one or more of the complicating disease mechanisms discussed above while at the same time having a pronounced candidicidal effect. The chart on the following pages shows a comparison of some of these and the issues each addresses. Of these, for women with candidiasis and infertility, I frequently chose to use *Er Xian Tang, Yang Wei Yi Qi Tang, Wen Jing Tang, Wu Mei Wan, Tao He Cheng Qi Tang*, and *Nei Yi Wan* as guiding formulas at least in Phase III. The first two of these formulas I use mostly for luteal phase defect and candidiasis, while the remaining four I use for candidiasis and endometriosis or uterine myoma.

Er Xian Tang is most commonly thought of as a menopausal prescription. However, Sun Ning-quan's luteal phase defect protocol discussed in Chapter 5 can be seen as a modified *Er Xian Tang*.

Rx: *Er Xian Tang*

Rhizoma Anemarrhenae (*Zhi Mu*)
Cortex Phellodendri (*Huang Bai*)
Radix Morindae Officinalis (*Ba Ji Tian*)
Rhizoma Curculiginis Orchoidis (*Xiao Mao*)
Herba Epimedii (*Xian Ling Pi*)
Radix Angelicae Sinensis (*Dang Gui*)

Based on the above considerations of candidiasis and damp heat playing a role in progesterone deficiency early periods accompanied by symptoms of hyperestrogenosis, I often use Sun's protocol with the addition of Rhizoma Anemarrhenae (*Zhi Mu*) and Cortex Phellodendri (*Huang Bai*). Of the remaining ingredients, I often delete

Damp Heat & Its Complications
Of Spleen Vacuity, Kidney Yin Vacuity,
Kidney Yang Vacuity,
Cold Below, & Blood Stasis

Upper Burner	Heat & Dryness Above	Heat Above	Heat & Dryness Above	Heat & Dryness Above	Dryness Above
Middle Burner	Spleen Vacuity Dampness	Spleen Vacuity			
Lower Burner	Cold Below Blood Stasis	Cold Below Blood Stasis	Cold Below Blood Stasis Heat entering *xue fen*	Damp Heat entering *xue fen*	Cold Below Damp Heat Blood Stasis
Rx	*Wen Jing Tang*	*Wu Mei Wan*	*Tao He Cheng Qi Tang*	*Wen Qing Yin, San Huang Si Wu Tang*	*Yi Yi Fu Zi Bai Jiang San*

	Heat & Dryness Above		Heat Above	Heat & Dryness Above	Heat & Dryness Above
	Spleen Vacuity Qi Vacuity	Spleen Vacuity	Spleen Vacuity		
Damp Heat Below	Damp Heat	Summer Heat Invasion (i.e., Damp Heat Below)	Damp Heat	Yin Vacuity Damp Heat Below	Yin & Yang Vacuity Damp Heat Below
Bai Tou Weng Tang, Ge Geng Huang Qin Huang Lian Tang, Long Dan Xie Gan Tang	*Dang Gui Niu Huang Tang, Lian Zi Qing Xin Yin, Qing Re Yang Yin San*	*Huo Xiang Zheng Qi Tang*	*Ban Xia Xie Xin Tang, Sheng Jiang Xie Xin Tang, Gan Cao Xie Xin Tang, Gui Zhi Tang, He Xiang Lian Wan*	*Zhi Bai Di Huang Wan*	*Er Xian Tang, Gui Fu Di Huang Tang Jia Jian, Zi Shen Tong Guan Wan*

and substitute other appropriate medicinals for the Radix Linderae Strychnifoliae (*Wu Yao*) and Rhizoma Alismatis (*Ze Xie*) depending upon the individual case.

Frequently, I combine the main kidney-supplementing ingredients of *Er Xian Tang* with the main ingredients of *Huang Qi Ren Shen Tang*, Li Dong-yuan's formula.

Rx: *Huang Qi Ren Shen Tang*

Radix Astragali Membranacei (*Huang Qi*)
Radix Panacis Ginseng (*Ren Shen*)
Rhizoma Cimicifugae (*Sheng Ma*)
Cortex Phellodendri (*Huang Bai*)
Rhizoma Atractylodis Macrocephalae (*Bai Zhu*)
Rhizoma Atractylodis (*Cang Zhu*)
mix-fried Radix Glycyrrhizae (*Zhi Gan Cao*)
Tuber Ophiopogonis Japonicae (*Mai Dong*)
Radix Angelicae Sinensis (*Dang Gui*)
Pericarpium Citri Reticulatae (*Chen Pi*)
Massa Medica Fermentata (*Shen Qu*)
Fructus Schizandrae Chinensis (*Wu Wei Zi*)

This formula is a very sophisticated one for clearing both vacuity heat above and damp heat below, supplementing the heart, spleen, and kidney qi, rectifying the *chong mai*, *du mai*, and *ren mai*, and promoting ascension of the clear and descension of the turbid, thus automatically rectifying the qi. Commonly, I delete the last two ingredients and then add Rhizoma Curculiginis Orchoidis and Herba Epimedii from *Er Xian Tang* above. The resulting formula is even more effective for supplementing *jing* essence and warming the uterus while boosting and rectifying the qi and clearing and eliminating dampness and heat. Readers are referred to *Li Dong-yuan's Treatise on the Spleen & Stomach, A Translation of the Pi Wei Lun* for further insight into the modifications of his formula and Li's theories concerning yin fire and the *chong mai*.

In some cases, I may use a modification of *Er Xian Tang* up until the day before the period and then switch to *Wen Jing Tang* if there is dysmenorrhea with diarrhea, nausea, and chilled extremities following Li Heng-you's example of treating *gong han* or cold uterus. It is also possible to combine these two formulas as Ted Kaptchuk has demonstrated in his patent formula, Women's Journey. However, in infertility and endometriosis I would pick somewhat different ingredients, since Dr. Kaptchuk's formula is more designed to treat menopausal hot flashes and headaches.

Wu Mei Wan is the classical representative antiparasitic formula in TCM. However, I have treated a number of cases of intractable dysmenorrhea and endometriosis complicated by candidiasis with this formula. Some modifications for this formula used in treating abdominal pain are given above in Chapter 8. When it works, it can be amazingly effective. It was Cao and Tang's suggestion of this formula for chronic endometriosis with a mixture of hot and cold and my own ideas about candidiasis being a species of *chong* which led me to experiment with this formula. When it worked so astonishingly in several cases of previously recalcitrant dysmenorrhea and endometriosis, it led me to analyzing this formula's ingredients over and over again, and this has led me to clarify a number of issues on prescribing for patient's with PSCC.

Tao He Cheng Qi Tang also contains a combination of bitter, cold and acrid, warm ingredients and treats simultaneous heat and blood stasis with vacuity cold below. Although some practitioners may think that this formula can only be used in patients with constipation, if the Radix Et Rhizoma Rhei (*Da Huang*) is decocted with the other ingredients, its precipitating functions are reduced while it still retains its candidicidal properties along with its ability to crack long-standing stasis. To me, the key to this prescription is the combination of Radix

Et Rhizoma Rhei with Ramulus Cinnamomi (*Gui Zhi*) in terms of its treatment of candidiasis. Then the Semen Pruni Persicae (*Tao Ren*) combines with Radix Et Rhizoma Rhei to crack stasis and dispel stagnation. When other ingredients are added to these basic three, this too can be a very effective premenstrual or menstrual formula with women with candidiasis, endometriosis, and infertility. In this case, although there is an element of coldness and kidney vacuity present, heat and stasis predominate.

If there is no cold below but only dampness and heat and blood stasis complicated by kidney yin vacuity and heat and dryness above, I sometimes also use a modern experimental formula for endometriosis called *Nei Yi Wan*. It is composed of three ingredients:

Radix Et Rhizoma Rhei (*Da Huang*)
Carapax Amydae (*Bie Jia*)
Succinum (*Hu Po*)

As we have seen above, Radix Et Rhizoma Rhei not only cracks and dispels old, chronic stasis and clears heat from the intestines, it is also strongly antimycotic. Succinum is often thought of as a spirit calming medicinal. However, it also disinhibits urination in cases of damp heat urinary disturbance and quickens the blood, disperses swelling. Carapax Amydae is typically first thought of as a yin supplement and harnesser of ascendant yang, yet it also quickens the blood and disinhibits menstruation, scatters nodulation and cools the blood. Thus this formula treats dampness and heat binding with stasis below, an element of yin vacuity with heat in the blood, and heat and dryness above.

In many contemporary protocols for endometriosis, medicinals derived from tree sap or gum as blood-quickening ingredients are advised. These include Gummum Olibani (*Ru Xiang*), Myrrha (*Mo Yao*), Sanguis Draconis (*Xue Jie*), and Succinum (*Hu Po*). Since Succinum also disinhibits urination and thus indirectly clears heat from the lower burner, this ingredient seems especially appropriate

where candidiasis, heat inversion of the *chong mai*, damp heat below
and vexatious heat above are involved with endometriosis. The other
three sap ingredients all equally quicken the blood, transform stasis,
and generate new tissue. But only the Succinum specifically addresses
a component of damp heat below and vexatious heat above.

In China, *Nei Yi Wan* is sometimes given alone as an experimental
treatment for endometriosis. In the treatment of uterine myoma, its
three ingredients are often combined with other blood-quickening,
stasis-transforming medicinals. Personally, I never prescribe this trio
alone. However, I have found it to be a very effective and subtle
combination when treating endometriosis and myomas. For instance,
I have sometimes combined this formula with *Huang Qi Ren Shen
Tang* above to good effect in the treatment of endometriosis.

The above formulas are only some suggestions. Keeping these in
mind, one can return to the modern Chinese fertility protocols
described in Chapters 4-9 and modify these in the light of the above
discussions on candidiasis and medicinals which are useful in the
treatment of this condition. However, please let me be clear on one
point. I am not suggesting that all cases of female infertility involve
candidiasis nor that, when there is candidiasis, all one has to do is
employ antifungal medicinals to *sha jun* or kill microbes.

What I am saying is that chronic candidiasis often plays a part in
women's infertility and other endocrine dyscrasias. When one takes
this into account, it helps explain the Western biological mechanisms
of numerous Chinese medicinals and formulas. It can also help
modify and customize various formulas and protocols to more
effectively treat our Western patient population. Still, for me as a
practitioner of TCM, the best gift this system of medicine has to offer
the Western world is its method of predicating treatment on the basis
of an individualized pattern discrimination. Taking candidiasis into
account along with Li Dong-yuan's theories on yin fire simply help
to more accurately and comprehensively parse out the various factors

in our typically complicated patients' cases. Thus, taking candidiasis into consideration when making a TCM diagnosis and writing a TCM prescription should only make one's treatment based on pattern discrimination all the more accurate and, therefore, effective.

11

Special Difficulties Treating Infertility with TCM in the West & Some Personal Observations

Although TCM typically treats chronic, functional diseases as well if not better than and certainly cheaper and with less side effects than modern Western medicine, the TCM treatment of female infertility here in the United States is made difficult by at least two leading complicating factors. The first is that, in the West, female infertility as suggested above is very much related to delaying childbirth past the time when fertility naturally diminishes with age. Most women seeking treatment for infertility at my clinic are older than *most* of the women described in the Chinese research protocols in the chapters above. This means that treatment must typically last longer and often requires higher doses of medicinals. This leads directly to the second difficulty.

Because TCM in the West is not currently incorporated into the delivery system of socialized medicine, women must pay for their TCM medicinals out of their own pockets. Chinese herbs are relatively expensive for an alternative therapy for a non life-threatening condition. This means that our patients often cannot or will not pay for the full doses as used in the People's Republic of China. Although I have chosen not to give the exact amounts per ingredient in the formulas and protocols recorded in this book, I can say that the doses in modern Chinese fertility protocols are typically higher than in formulas for many other diseases. Commonly, each ingredient is listed at 12–15 grams apiece rather than the more standard 9 grams

239

apiece. I, for instance, feel I must prescribe my American patients half the normal TCM doses used in China due to the herbs' relatively high cost. Even still, my patients may have to spend $3-5 per day on these medicinals for many months on end.

When these difficulties are coupled with a racing biological clock and the lack of true trust and belief of Western patients in Eastern treatments, it can be very difficult to encourage a woman to stay with the program long enough to achieve her so fervently desired goal. In addition, other therapies may offer competing solutions which tempt our patients away from us, offering them supposedly quicker, surer results. This is especially so in the case of modern Western medicine whose doctors still occupy a role in the community bordering on that of a priest of an orthodox religion. For the vast majority of our patients in the West, modern Western medicine is what is really real.

Therefore, in order to gain long term compliance, it is, in my experience, of utmost importance to explain to the patient their TCM diagnosis and treatment plan. Further, the patient should be alerted to all the changes initiated by her TCM therapy which suggest she is moving toward her goal. These may include more and fresher looking menstrual blood, less cramps and clots, a better biphasic BBT curve, on time menstruation, and less PMS. All of these changes should confirm for the patient that 1) she is getting systemically healthier and 2) according to the theory and practice of TCM, she is increasing her fertility.

It is also extremely important that the practitioner counsel infertility patients on diet, stress reduction, and exercise as essential components in their total treatment plan. Without proper diet according to the principles of TCM dietary therapy, one cannot expect a satisfactory result from the herbs alone. In particular, diet plays a dominant role in women suffering from candidiasis and hyperimmune or allergic states. It is also crucially important in women with PMS. I have written at length on the relationship of diet to PMS in *PMS: Its Cause,*

Diagnosis & Treatment According to Traditional Chinese Medicine.[1] Similarly, stress reduction is vitally important in all women with either yin vacuity or liver qi. This accounts for a very large segment of our Western infertility patient population. Without programmed, daily, deep relaxation and stress reduction, such women must be counseled that they can hardly expect a totally satisfactory result from taking the Chinese herbs alone. And for anyone with either phlegm and dampness, liver qi and blood stasis, or insufficiency of qi and blood, regular exercise is also extremely important. At our clinic, we call these the three free therapies and all patients are required to have a one hour consultation on their implementation as part of their total treatment plan. I have written about the rationale and specifics of their implementation in numerous other places.

Likewise, some women, in their desire to do everything they possibly can in the shortest period of time, will also desire to receive regular acupuncture treatment in tandem with Chinese herbal therapy. In China, TCM *fu ke* specialists only prescribe traditional Chinese medicinals. Here in the West, the vast majority of TCM practitioners are trained and licensed primarily as acupuncturists. If a practitioner only has access to patent pills and desiccated extracts, combining herbal medicine and acupuncture on a routine basis makes sense, since I do not believe the doses of these are sufficient for the majority of older women seeking treatment for infertility. In addition, one may not have the ability to modify their formulas as carefully as necessary using such pills and powders and, therefore, acupuncture may be used to amplify and extend the effects of those medicaments. However, if one dispenses bulk herbs in relatively strong doses, regular acupuncture treatments may make the total cost of treatment prohibitively expensive considering that most Western patients are only "trying" Chinese medicine. Because treatment for infertility in the West must so commonly be given over a protracted period of

---

[1] Flaws, Bob, *PMS: Its Cause, Diagnosis & Treatment According to Traditional Chinese Medicine*, Blue Poppy Press, Boulder, CO, 1991

241

time, I typically do not advise or require regularly scheduled acupuncture. Rather, I have my patients put their money into the herbal medicine itself and make sure they understand how to implement the three free therapies above.

I know that many Western practitioners feel that Chinese herbal medicine in decoction is inappropriate for Westerners. According to this point of view, it is difficult and time-consuming to prepare, tastes bad, and compliance is low. However, it is no more time-consuming or labor intensive than cooking a pot of rice and can be done when making dinner. If one does not have time to make their own dinner each night, that in itself is a problem. The herbs taste bad only initially or when the prescription is erroneous, remembering that bad is a subjective judgement. Coffee tastes equally as bitter as most Chinese herbal decoctions, yet many people love its taste. If the prescription is correct, the "bad" taste disappears within 36-72 hours and the patient will even come to crave their medicine or, at the very least, not mind taking it.

In my experience, compliance is only an issue in the majority of Western patients if the practitioner likewise has a problem with bulk herbs in decoction. When patients come to me, they know ahead of time that I specialize in TCM gynecology and that the main modality of TCM gynecology is drinking bitter tasting Chinese herbal decoctions. They know this either by word of mouth or my receptionist is clear in explaining this. Therefore, my prescription of Chinese herbs in decoction is not an option. It is simply standard operating procedure. Since I drink Chinese herbal medicine in decoction on a pretty regular basis and have no problems with it, neither do the majority of my patients. More and more, I see that how the therapist thinks and feels about their therapy colors their patients' reactions to it, even when those thoughts and feelings are not overtly communicated to the patient.

Timing Conception While Taking Chinese Herbal Medicine

Very commonly, women will ask what effects their herbs will have on their pregnancy and their child if they conceive at midcycle and then take herbs until later in the month when it becomes apparent that they have conceived. I have heard that some practitioners counsel their patients not to even attempt to conceive until after all their signs and symptoms suggest that they can. At that point, they are told to stop their medication and see what happens.

I too agree that, for emotional reasons, women should be counseled not to attempt to conceive until their signs and symptoms significantly improve. This is not to protect the fetus but to protect the mother against the roller-coaster of hope, anticipation, elation, and depression which so many women experience every cycle when they are trying to conceive. Because of the relationship between the hypothalamus, the pituitary, and the ovaries or between the kidneys, the liver, and the qi and blood, if you will, this cycle of anticipation and depression causes internal damage due to the seven passions. In Chinese, this is called *qi qing nei shang*. As we have seen above, many Chinese doctors, both classical and contemporary, believe that stress plays a very large, negative role in most women's infertility. Thus avoidance of such emotional ups and downs is important if this negative factor affecting their fertility is to be eliminated.

The fear that some practitioners have is that blood-quickening medicinals taken after the time of conception may actually induce a spontaneous abortion. However, I do not think that this is the case. Infertile women with liver qi commonly have a luteal phase defect. Because of this qi stagnation, they may already be conceiving and miscarrying month after month. It is the rectification of the qi and quickening of the blood which actually remedies this condition. Such qi-rectification and blood quickening is often spoken of in Chinese under the abbreviation, *tiao jing*, regulating the menses. Therefore, I do not advise such women not to try to conceive when they are taking qi-rectifying, blood-quickening medicinals for fear of causing an abortion. Once the period is overdue, then I recommend the patient to do a home pregnancy test. If she is pregnant, that is when I reconsider the formula she is on.

However, in my experience, women with liver qi and a luteal phase defect who have had trouble conceiving, also have trouble maintaining the pregnancy *because* of remaining liver qi. In this case, these women may experience lower abdominal pain during pregnancy which, in TCM, is a possible premonitory sign of spontaneous abortion. In these women, it is rectifying the qi, quickening the blood, and relieving depression which save the pregnancy. In such cases, such therapy does not cause but actually prevents miscarriage.

For sure, qi-moving, blood-quickening medicinals will aggravate a woman's condition and may lead to a miscarriage if they are erroneously given to a vacuous and insufficient woman. This underscores the importance of prescribing on the basis of a *bian zheng* diagnosis. If one desires to use one of the disease-based protocols above, it is my strong conviction and advice that one should only use a protocol whose ingredients also conform to the patient's individualized TCM pattern diagnosis. When one proceeds in this manner, one should never be administering treatment which is too strong or inappropriate for the patient at any phase of their cycle whether they have conceived or not.

Tracking Ovulation by the Ferning of the Oral Mucous

Although charting the BBT gives a good idea of, if, and when ovulation occurs, there is another way to corroborate ovulation. Women's mucous becomes crystalline in reaction to progesterone. In the vagina, the crystallization of the vaginal mucous gives rise to the tacky, sticky mucous known as spin mucous. Informed Choice of Campbell, CA markets a plastic lens for $29.95. With this lens, a woman can observe the characteristic crystallization or ferning pattern of her mucous, revealed under magnification. Since all mucous in the body displays this ferning pattern in reaction to progesterone, the woman can easily see this by magnifying a drop of her oral mucous.

This easy and inexpensive method of verifying if and when ovulation has taken place can not only help time changes in TCM herbal therapy but can also provide emotional support for women needing to be reassured they are ovulating. The address of Informed Choice is 1191 Ridgeley, Campbell, CA 95008 and their phone number is 1-800-723-0400.

BIBLIOGRAPHY

Chinese Sources

Bai Ling Fu Ke (Bai-ling's Gynecology), Han Bai-ling, Heilongjiang Peoples Press, Harbin, 1983

Fu Ke Bing (Gynecological Diseases), California Certified Acupuncturists Association, Oakland, CA, 1988

Fu Ke Bing Liang Fang (Fine Formulas for Gynecological Diseases), He Yuan-lin & Jiang Chang-yun, Yunnan University Press, Chongqing, 1991

Fu Ke Lin Chuan Jing Hua (The Clinical Essence of Gynecology), Wang Bu-ru & Wang Qi-ming, Sichuan Science & Technology Press, Cheng-du, 1989

Fu Ke San Bai Zheng (Three Hundred Gynecological Conditions), Liu Lan-fang & Liu Dian-gong, Jiangxi Science & Technology Press, 1989

Fu Ke Yu Chi (The Jade Rule of Gynecology), Shen Jin-ao, Shanghai Science & Technology Press, Shanghai, 1983

Fu Ke Zheng Zhi (Proven Treatments in Gynecology), Sun Jiu-ling, Hebei Peoples Press, 1983

Fu Qing Zhu Nu Ke (Fu Qing-zhu's Gynecology), Fu Qing-zhu, Shanghai Peoples Press, Shanghai, 1979; available in English, trans. by Yang Shou-zhong & Liu Da-wei, Blue Poppy Press, Boulder, CO, 1992

Fu Ren Da Quan Liang Fang (A Large Collection of Fine Formulas for Women), Chen Ze-ming, Peoples Government Press, Beijing, 1985

Han Ying Chang Yong Yi Xue Ci Hui (Chinese-English Glossary of Commonly Used Medical Terms), Huang Xiao-kai, Peoples Health & Hygeine Press, Beijing, 1982

Nu Ke Bai Wen (100 Questions on Gynecology), Qi Chong-fu, Shanghai Ancient Chinese Medical Books Press, Shanghai, 1983

Nu Ke Ji Yao (The Collected Essentials of Gynecology), Yu Yao-feng, Peoples Government Press, Beijing, 1988

Nu Ke Mi Jue Da Quan (Complete Secrets of Success in Gynecology), Chen Liang-fang, Beijing Daily Press, Beijing, 1989

Nu Ke Xian Fang (Immortal Formulas in Gynecology), Fu Shan, aka Fu Qing-zhu, Ancient Chinese Medical Book Press, Beijing, 1989

Nu Ke Yao Zhi (The Essentials of Gynecology), Yu Yo-yuan, Fujian Science & Technology Press, Fuzhou, 1982

Nan Nu Bing Mi Yan Liang Fang (Secret, Proven, Fine Formulas for Men's & Women's Disease), Du Jie-hui, Beijing Science & Technology press, Beijing, 1991

Shang Hai Lao Zhong Yi Jing Yan Xuan Bian (A Selected Compilation of Shanghai Old Doctors' Experiences), Shanghai Science & Technology Press, Shanghai, 1984

Shi Yong Zhong Xi Yi Jie He Fu Chan Ke Zheng Zhi (Proven Treatments in Practical Integrated Chinese-Western Obstetrics & Gynecology), Guo Yuan, Shanxi Peoples Press, Xian, 1984

Wan Shi Fu Ren Ke (Master Wan's Gynecology), Wan Quan, aka

Wan Mi-zhai, Hubei Science & Technology Press, 1984

Yi Zong Jin Jian (The Golden Mirror of Ancestral Medicine), Wu Qian *et al.*, Peoples Health & Hygeine Press, Beijing, 1985

Yu Xue Zheng Zhi (Proven Treatments for Blood Stasis), Zhang Xue-wen, Shanxi Science & Technology Press, Xian, 1986

Zhong Yi Fu Chan Ke Xue (The Study of Chinese Medical Gynecology and Obstetrics), Heilonjiang College of TCM, People's Health and Hygiene Press, Beijing, 1991

Zhong Yi Fu Ke (Traditional Chinese Gynecology), Zhu Cheng-han, Peoples Heath & Hygeine Press, Beijing, 1989

Zhong Yi Fu Ke Lin Chuan Shou Ce (A Handbook of Clinical TCM Gynecology), Shen Chong-li, Shanghai Science & Technology Press, Shanghai, 1990

Zhong Yi Fu Ke Shou Ce (A Handbook of Traditional Chinese Gynecology), Song Guang-ji & Yu Xiao-zhen, Zhejiang Science & Technology Press, Hangzhou, 1984; available in English, second, revised edition, trans. by Zhang Ting-liang & Bob Flaws, Blue Poppy Press, Boulder, CO, 1991

Zhong Yi Fu Ke Xue (A Study of TCM Gynecology), Chengdu College of TCM, Shanghai Science & Technology Press, Shanghai, 1983

Zhong Yi Fu Ke Xue (The Study of TCM Gynecology), Luo Yuan-qi, Shanghai Science & Technology Press, Shanghai, 1987

Zhong Yi Fu Ke Zhi Liao Shou Ce (A Handbook of TCM Gynecological Treatment), Wu Shi-xing & Qi Cheng-lin, Shan Xi Science & Technology Press, Xian, 1991

Zhong Yi Hu Li Xue (A Study of TCM Nursing), Lu Su-ying, Peoples Health & Hygeine Press, Beijing, 1983

Zhong Yi Lin Chuang Ge Ke (Various Clinical Specialties in TCM), Zhang En-qin *et al.*, Shanghai College of TCM Press, Shanghai, 1990

Zhong Yi Zhi Liao Fu Ke Bing (The TCM Treatment of Gynecological Diseases), Zhang Jian-xiu, Hebei Science & Technology Press, 1988

English Sources

A Barefoot Doctor's Manual, revised & enlarged edition, Cloudburst Press, Mayne Isle, 1977

A Clinical Guide to Chinese Herbs and Formulae, Cheng Song-yu & Li Fei, Churchill & Livingstone, Edinburgh, 1993

A Comprehensive Guide to Chinese Herbal Medicine, Chen Ze-lin & Chen Mei-fang, Oriental Healing Arts Institute, Long Beach, CA, 1992

Chinese-English Terminology of Traditional Chinese Medicine, Shuai Xue-zhong *et al.*, Hunan Science & Technology Press, Changsha, 1983

Chinese-English Manual of Common-used Prescriptions in Traditional Chinese Medicine, Ou Ming, ed., Joint Publishing Co., Ltd., Hong Kong, 1989

Chinese Herbal Medicine: Formulas & Strategies, Dan Bensky & Randall Barolet, Eastland Press, Seattle, 1990

Chinese Herbal Medicine: Materia Medica, Dan Bensky & Andrew Gamble, Eastland, Press, Seattle, 1986

Chinese Materia Medica, Vol. 1-6, Southern Materials Center, Inc, Taipei, 1979

Concise Traditional Chinese Gynecology, Xia Gui-cheng *et al.*, Jiangsu Science & Technology Press, Nanjing, 1988

Fundamentals of Chinese Medicine, Nigel Wiseman & Andrew Ellis, Paradigm Publications, Brookline, MA, 1985

Glossary of Chinese Medical Terms and Acupuncture Points, Nigel Wiseman & Ken Boss, Paradigm Publications, Brookline, MA, 1990

Handbook of Chinese Herbs and Formulas, Him-che Yeung, self-published, LA, 1985

Illustrated Differentiations of Syndromes and Treatment for Internal Injury Diseases, Huang Bing-shan, self-published, Denver, CO, 1990

Intractable Dysmenorrhea: Experiences of Master Physicians Shen Long Li and Ma Long Bai, trans. by C.S. Cheung, Harmonious Sunshine Cultural Center, Sunnyvale, CA, 1988

Orienal Materia Medica, A Concise Guide, Hong-yen Hsu, Oriental Healing Arts Institute, Long Beach, CA, 1986

Practical Traditional Chinese Medicine & Pharmacology: Clinical Experiences, Shang Xian-min *et al.*, New World Press, Beijing, 1990

Practical Traditional Chinese Medicine & Pharmacology: Herbal Formulas, Geng Jun-ying, *et al.*, New World Press, Beijing, 1991

The English-Chinese Encyclopedia of Practical Traditional Chinese

Medicine, Vol. 12: Gynecology, Xuan Jia-sheng, ed., Higher Education Press, Beijing, 1990

The Essential Book of Traditional Chinese Medicine, Vol. 2: Clinical Practice, Liu Yan-chi, trans. by Fang Ting-yu & Chen Lai-di, Columbia University Press, NY, 1988

The Merck Manual, 15th edition, ed. by Robert Berkow, Merck Sharp & Dohme Research Laboratories, Rahway, NJ, 1987

The Yeast Connection, William G. Crook, Vintage Books, Random House, New York, 1986

The Yeast Syndrome, John Parks Towbridge & Morton Walker, Bantam Books, Toronto, 1988

Traditional Chinese Medicine: Handbook (of) Differential Diagnosis (&) Treatment, Vol. 1-3, Ou-yang Yi, trans. by C.S. Cheung, Harmonious Sunshine Cultural Center, San Francisco, 1987

Traditional Medicine in Contemporary China, Nathan Sivin, University of Michigan, Ann Arbor, 1987

Zang Fu: The Organ Systems of Traditional Chinese Medicine, second edition, Jeremy Ross, Churchill Livingstone, Edinburgh, 1985

General Index

A

A Handbook of Clinical TCM Gynecology 28
A Handbook of TCM Gynecological Treatment 36, 41
A Handbook of Traditional Chinese Urology & Male Sexual Dysfunction 209
A Study of TCM Gynecology & Obstetrics 42, 49, 70
abdomen, chilly pain in the lower 34, 72, 77
abdomen, lumps inside the 196
abdomen, stabbing pain in the lower 91
abdominal pain aggravated as the period draws near 91
abdominal pain ameliorated by warmth 73
abdominal pain, severe 65, 191
abdominal pain with the arrival of the menses accompanied by fever 190
abortions 16
accumulation and gathering 201
acne 221
acupuncture 21, 241
Addison's disease 218
adhesions 7, 8, 155, 164, 169, 203
adnexitis 170
adrenal hyperplasia 2, 109
agglutination of the mucosal folds 155
aging 11, 16
alimentary tract 214
allergic reaction 6, 217, 218, 227, 230
allergies, atopic 212
allergies, food 218, 221
allergies, sperm 210
alopecia 218
amenorrhea 26, 51, 70, 80, 97, 103, 106, 107, 138-140, 146, 175, 176, 182, 183, 219

anally administered medicinals 169
anemia, pernicious 152, 218
angered, easily 59, 64, 153
anovulation 20, 23, 95, 106, 109, 121, 138-140, 175
anovulation, chronic 175
antibiotics 8, 217
antibodies, agglutinating 6
antiovarian antibodies 216
APICH 217, 219, 221
appetite, poor 129
arthritis, rheumatoid 152, 219
attacking therapies 157
autism 219
autoimmune factors 152

B

bacteria 8, 214, 215
bao gong 19, 26
bao luo 92, 167
basal body temperature 5, 6, 96, 97, 137, 168
basal body temperature, abnormalities in 97
BBT 5, 6, 97-100, 104-106, 115, 137, 143, 172, 229, 230, 240, 244
Bei Run-pu 167, 169
belching 59, 221
Ben Cao Gang Mu 159
Bensky and Barolet 56, 57, 79
bian zheng lun zhi 8, 21, 22, 25
biological clock 240
biopsy 7, 137
biphasic graph 6
bitter, cold medicinals 225, 230
bleeding, irregular, profuse uterine 175
bleeding, midcycle 96, 109, 133, 135, 148, 152, 182
bleeding, pathologic 17
bloating 221

Formula Index

A, B

Ai Fu Nuan Gong Wan 77
Ba Sheng Dan 46
Ba Zhen Yi Mu Wan 56
Bai Ling Tiao Gan Tang 59
Bao Luo Hua Yu Tang Jia Jian 92
Bu Shen Fang 139
Bu Shen Hua Shi Tang 82
Bu Shen Qing Re Fang 150
Bu Shen Shu Gan Fang 139
Bu Shen Shu Yu Tang 142
Bu Shen Si Wu Tang 146
Bu Zhong Yi Qi Tang 87, 193
Bu Zhong Yi Qi Tang Jia Wei 87

C

Cang Fu Dao Tan Wan 82, 84, 176
Cang Fu Dao Tan Wan Jia Jian #1 83
Cang Fu Dao Tan Wan Jia Jian #2 83
Cang Zhu Dao Tan Wan Jia Wei 85
Chai Hu Shu Gan San 60
Cu Huang Ti Tang 145, 148, 180
Cu Luan Bao Tang 124, 179

D

Dan Zhi Xiao Yao San Jia Gu Jing
  Wan 52
Dang Gui Jian Zhong Tang 192
Dang Gui Shao Yao San 57
Dang Gui Yang Xue Tang Jia Wei 58
De Sheng Tang Jia Wei 62

E, F

Er Chen Wan 86
Er Si Wu He Ji 30, 32
Er Xian Tang Jia Jian 37

Fu Ke Bing Liang Fang 32
Fu Ke Lin Chuang Jing Hua 84
Fu Ke San Bai Zheng 61
Fu Zi Li Zhong Wan 192

G, H

Gu Yin Jian 210, 211
Gui Pi Wan 126
Gui Zhi Fu Ling Wan 75, 76, 194
Gui Zhi Fu Ling Wan Jia Wei 75
Hong Teng Er Hao Fang 165, 166
Hong Teng Yi Hao Fang 165, 166
Huang Qi Jian Zhong Tang 192
Huang Qi Ren Shen Tang 234, 237
Huo Xue Tiao Jing Tang 181

J, K

Ji Kun Da Zao Wan 46
Jia Jian Chai Hu Shu Gan San 60
Jia Jian Shao Fu Zhu Yu Tang 71
Jia Jian Wen Shen Wan 36
Jia Jian Zuo Gui Wan 29
Jia Wei Di Huang Tang 42
Jia Wei Fu Ling Wan 195
Jia Wei Qi Gong Wan 81
Jia Wei Xiao Yao San 59
Jian Quon Huang Ti Tang 147
Jin Gui Shen Qi Wan 35
Jin Lian Zhong Zi Fang 37
Kai Yu Zhong Yu Tang 61, 72, 128
Kai Yu Zhong Yu Tang Jia Jian 72
Kuan Dai Tang 40

L

Liang Di Tang Jia Wei 48
Liu Wei Di Huang Tang Jia Jian 43
Liu Wei Di Huang Wan Jia Jian 116

265

OTHER BOOKS ON CHINESE MEDICINE
AVAILABLE FROM
BLUE POPPY PRESS

1775 Linden Ave
Boulder, CO 80304
For ordering 1-800-487-9296
PH. 303\447-8372 FAX 303\447-0740

PMS: Its Cause, Diagnosis & Treatment According to Traditional Chinese Medicine by Bob Flaws ISBN 0-936185-22-8 $14.95

SOMETHING OLD, SOMETHING NEW; Essays on the TCM Description of Western Herbs, Pharmaceuticals, Vitamins & Minerals by Bob Flaws ISBN 0-936185-21-X $19.95

SCATOLOGY & THE GATE OF LIFE: The Role of the Large Intestine in Immunity, An Integrated Chinese-Western Approach by Bob Flaws ISBN 0-936185-20-1 $12.95

SECOND SPRING: A Guide To Healthy Menopause Through Traditional Chinese Medicine by Honora Lee Wolfe ISBN 0-936185-18-X $14.95

MIGRAINES & TRADITIONAL CHINESE MEDICINE: A Layperson's Guide by Bob Flaws ISBN 0-936185-15-5 $11.95

STICKING TO THE POINT: A Rational Methodology for the Step by Step Formulation & Administration of an Acupuncture Treatment by Bob Flaws ISBN 0-936185-17-1 $14.95

ENDOMETRIOSIS & INFERTILITY AND TRADITIONAL CHINESE MEDICINE: A Laywoman's Guide by Bob Flaws ISBN 0-936185-14-7 $9.95

THE BREAST CONNECTION: A Laywoman's Guide to the Treatment of Breast Disease by Chinese Medicine by Honora Lee Wolfe ISBN 0-936185-13-9 $8.95

NINE OUNCES: A Nine Part Program For The Prevention of AIDS in HIV Positive Persons by Bob Flaws ISBN 0-936185-12-0 $9.95

THE TREATMENT OF CANCER BY INTEGRATED

CHINESE-WESTERN
MEDICINE by Zhang Dai-
zhao, trans. by Zhang Ting-liang
ISBN 0-936185-11-2 $16.95

A HANDBOOK OF
TRADITIONAL CHINESE
DERMATOLOGY by Liang
Jian-hui, trans. by Zhang Ting-
liang & Bob Flaws, ISBN 0-
936185-07-4 $14.95

A HANDBOOK OF
TRADITIONAL CHINESE
GYNECOLOGY by Zhejiang
College of TCM, trans. by Zhang
Ting-liang, ISBN 0-936185-06-6
(2nd edit.) $21.95

FREE & EASY: Traditional
Chinese Gynecology for
American Women 2nd Edition,
by Bob Flaws, ISBN 0-936185-
05-8 $15.95

PRINCE WEN HUI'S
COOK: Chinese Dietary
Therapy by Bob Flaws &
Honora Lee Wolfe, ISBN 0-
912111-05-4, $12.95 (Published by
Paradigm Press, Brookline, MA)

THE DAO OF
INCREASING LONGEVITY
AND CONSERVING ONE'S
LIFE by Anna Lin & Bob Flaws,
ISBN 0-936185-24-4 $16.95

FIRE IN THE VALLEY:
The TCM Diagnosis and
Treatment of Vaginal
Diseases by Bob Flaws
ISBN 0-936185-25-2 $16.95

HIGHLIGHTS OF
ANCIENT ACUPUNCTURE
PRESCRIPTIONS trans. by
Honora Lee Wolfe & Rose
Crescenz ISBN 0-936185-23-6
$14.95

ARISAL OF THE CLEAR:
A Simple Guide to Healthy
Eating According to
Traditional Chinese Medicine
by Bob Flaws, ISBN #-936185-
27-9 $8.95

CERVICAL DYSPLASIA &
PROSTATE CANCER:
HPV, A HIDDEN LINK? by
Bob Flaws, ISBN 0-936185-19-8
$23.95

PEDIATRIC BRONCHITIS:
ITS CAUSE, DIAGNOSIS &
TREATMENT
ACCORDING TO
TRADITIONAL CHINESE
MEDICINE trans. by Gao Yu-li
and Bob Flaws, ISBN 0-936185-
26-0 $15.95

AIDS & ITS TREATMENT
ACCORDING TO
TRADITIONAL CHINESE
MEDICINE by Huang Bing-
shan, trans. by Fu-Di & Bob
Flaws, ISBN 0-936185-28-7
$24.95

ACUTE ABDOMINAL
SYNDROMES: Their
Diagnosis & Treatment by
Combined Chinese-Western
Medicine by Alon Marcus, ISBN
0-936185-31-7 $16.95

BEFORE COMPLETION: Essays on the Practice of TCM by Bob Flaws, ISBN 0-936185-32-5, $16.95

MY SISTER, THE MOON: The Diagnosis & Treatment of Menstrual Diseases by Traditional Chinese Medicine by Bob Flaws, ISBN 0-936185-34-1, $24.95

FU QING-ZHU'S GYNECOLOGY trans. by Yang Shou-zhong and Liu Da-wei, ISBN 0-936185-35-X, $21.95

FLESHING OUT THE BONES: The Importance of Case Histories in Chinese Medicine trans. by Charles Chace. ISBN 0-936185-30-9, $18.95

CLASSICAL MOXIBUSTION SKILLS IN CONTEMPORARY CLINICAL PRACTICE by Sung Baek, ISBN 0-936185-16-3 $10.95

THE MEDICAL I CHING: Oracle of the Healer Within by Miki Shima, OMD, ISBN 0-936185-38-4, $19.95

MASTER TONG'S ACUPUNCTURE: An Ancient Lineage for Modern Practice, trans. and commentary by Miriam Lee, OMD, ISBN 0-936185-37-6, $19.95

A HANDBOOK OF TCM UROLOGY & MALE SEXUAL DYSFUNCTION by Anna Lin, OMD, ISBN 0-936185-36-8, $16.95

Li Dong-yuan's TREATISE ON THE SPLEEN & STOMACH, A Translation of the *Pi Wei Lun* by Yang Shou-zhong & Li Jian-yong, ISBN 0-936185-41-4, $21.95

PATH OF PREGNANCY, VOL. I, Gestational Disorders by Bob Flaws, ISBN 0-936185-39-2, $16.95

PATH OF PREGNANCY, VOL. II, Postpartum Diseases by Bob Flaws, ISBN 0-936185-42-2, $18.95

How to Have a HEALTHY PREGNANCY, HEALTHY BIRTH with Traditional Chinese Medicine by Honora Lee Wolfe, ISBN 0-936185-40-6, $9.95

MASTER HUA'S CLASSIC OF THE CENTRAL VISCERA by Hua Tuo, translated by Yang Shou-zhong, ISBN 0-936185-43-0, $21.95

A NEW AMERICAN ACUPUNCTURE: Acupuncture Osteopathy, by Mark Seem, ISBN 0-936185-44-9, $19.95

THE HEART & ESSENCE OF DAN-XI'S METHODS OF TREATMENT by Zhu Dan-xi, trans. by Yang Shou-zhong. ISBN 0-936185-50-3, $21.95

HOW TO WRITE A TCM HERBAL FORMULA A Logical Methodology for the Formulation & Administration of Chinese Herbal Medicine in Decoction, by Bob Flaws, ISBN 0-936185-49-X, $10.95